MW01075251

Adh
The Body's Hidden Menace
Is There a Cure?

by Larry Wurn, LMT and Belinda Wurn, PT

This book explores adhesions,
a hidden cause of chronic pain and dysfunction.

Adhesions are internal scars that can form in all people;
they can impact virtually every system in the body.

Printed in the United States of America
Copyright 2018 by Lawrence J Wurn
ISBN: 978-1986094788

For more information:
visit *www.clearpassage.com*
or email *info@clearpassage.com*

Table of Contents

Chapter 4
Adhesions and Chronic Pain............41

Chapter 5
Life-Threatening Intestinal Adhesions............56

CHAPTER 7
PUBLISHED DATA

Introduction

Background: At 32 years of age, Belinda was full of vitality. She had graduated physical therapy school *summa cum laude*, at the very top of her class. She was busy helping patients with serious physical conditions, and she had been certified to instruct physical therapy at the local medical school.

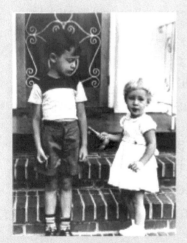

The authors share a happier time, years ago.

Belinda had remet the love of her life, a childhood friend who became a writer and a well-known figure in the San Francisco arts scene. They were planning their marriage when she received the awful diagnosis that changed her life.

"You have cancer," her physician said. "There is a tumor on your cervix at the entrance of your uterus. We need to address this aggressively and immediately."

Stunned but undaunted, she followed her doctor's advice to the letter. She had the surgery, then underwent 40 external radiation treatments to destroy the cancer cells. On two different occasions, she underwent 72 hours of internal radiation in a lead-lined room, where physicians placed radioactive material deep inside of her unprotected pelvis to help shrink and destroy the cancerous tumor.

The lead walls were designed to protect others who may be passing the room from being exposed to the radiation that we allowed them to place deeply into her body. "It's dangerous for any of us to be in the room for more than five minutes due to the radiation," the nurse explained. "But don't worry; we'll keep you deeply sedated."

"Looking back, it is hard to imagine we allowed Belinda to be exposed to so much radiation, but when you are facing cancer, and you have an esteemed team of physicians telling you this is what you must do to save your life, you tend to listen," her husband Larry said.

Belinda returned to work, determined to put the trauma and horror of those months behind her. "They got it all," she told her fiancé. "Let's get married and move on. It's time to create our lives and our family!"

Life was good again until a year later; Belinda began to have unexpected twinges, then stabbing pain deep in her pelvis. Concerned the cancer might be returning, she returned to her gynecologist for a checkup.

"The cancer is gone," her doctor said. "I hope that it will

not be coming back. Adhesions that your body created to help you heal from the radiation therapy and surgeries, are causing the pain. Hopefully, it will pass and won't affect your life much."

But it did affect her life. Over the next 12 months, the pain became so bad that it was debilitating. Belinda could not walk, move or even breathe without feeling deep, stabbing pains and a 'straitjacket' forming within the tissues of her pelvis. "I could feel it getting tighter over time," she said.

When she returned to her doctor, he said "There's nothing we can do about the pain; it has to be coming from the adhesions. They have formed in your delicate reproductive areas, your vagina and maybe your rectum. You certainly don't want us doing surgery there; that would only lead to more adhesions. We saved you from cancer. You will have to learn to live with the pain."

Belinda and Larry were stunned. With all of the advances in medical science, the cures for all the diseases that have plagued mankind over the centuries, and her esteemed team of expert physicians, how could it be that something as simple as tiny internal scars, actually caused by her doctors treatment, were giving her so much pain? Yet, no one could offer a cure.

Surely, there had to be an answer for Belinda. She and Larry consulted numerous physicians in their hometown, then across the state trying to find someone who could treat her adhesions. Gynecologists, neurologists, general surgeons, physical therapists – all accomplished and highly respected, yet none of them knew how to help Belinda find relief from her pain.

In frustration, the couple decided together "There has to be a way, even if we have to figure this out on our own."

Thus started a 30 year inquiry into adhesions, their structure, mechanism of formation, and a way to deform and detach them to return Belinda to a normal life. This book will summarize what they learned over those three decades. We will examine the reasons for the pain and dysfunction adhesions can cause, the conditions they affect, and what can be done about them.

-Larry Wurn

Chapter 1
What Are Adhesions?

From the first time we first fell and scraped our knee, a scar (called an adhesion) formed on the skin in the place where we healed. Long after healing has occurred, that scar remains on the surface of the skin, whether it's visible or not. In most cases, a surface scar or adhesion of this type is unlikely to cause any problems.

Now, remember when you were running or roller skating and you fell onto your bottom; or perhaps you hit the ground hard from the slide, or you fell off the climbing bars at the neighborhood park. If you landed on your tailbone (coccyx) and it became sufficiently bruised, tiny strands of collagen, the building blocks of adhesions, came rushing in to surround the area that was injured – to start the healing process. These strands cause *crosslinks*, powerful microscopic bonds that attach the collagen fiber to neighboring structures. Just like the scrape in your knee, these strands and crosslinks join together to form an adhesion at or beside your tailbone. Unless it dissipates in the first few days, that adhesion will generally remain there for your entire life.

If you are lucky, the adhesions remain on your coccyx

and don't affect neighboring structures. But if the trauma or inflammation from that fall was more severe, adhesions can spread to the ligaments that hold your tailbone in place.

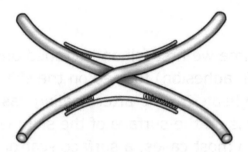

Adhesive crosslinks form as the first step in the healing process.

Like the ropes that hold a pup tent pole in place, the ligaments of the coccyx are designed to hold it in a perfectly aligned position. These ligaments allow your tailbone to move forward when you sit down, and to move back when you have a bowel movement or (for a woman) during intercourse. Adhesions from a fall can start to pull your coccyx forward or to one side.

As time goes by, the inflammation caused by successive pressure (e.g. from prolonged sitting during school years) on the already adhered ligaments can cause more inflammation; thus, more collagen crosslinks form to help the body continue to heal – but they now spread into nearby areas and structures.

By your late teens or early 20s, you may begin to notice digestive problems such as constipation, due to the tailbone being constantly pulled forward, partly closing the door to elimination of waste. You may notice difficulty sitting for long periods of time, perhaps even through a movie. If you are a sexually active woman, you may begin to experience pain with intercourse as your tailbone now sits in the way of deep penetration.

Headaches sometimes occur at the base of the skull due to the pull of the dura, which is the surrounding membrane of your spinal cord. As your forward tailbone pulls the entire spinal cord down, it can pull your head down onto the top of your cervical spine and cause pain in your neck, at the base of the skull or at the dural attachments within the cranium, such as the temples or the top of your head.

The forward pull of your tailbone and its resulting inability to fold back when necessary can cause problems in other areas. Since some tailbone ligaments attach directly into the hip, you may begin to experience pain in one or both hips, even years or decades after the original injury. If they spread to the nearby reproductive structures, infertility may result as adhesions squeeze the uterus or ovaries, or constrict the fallopian tube. Adhesions at the nearby bowel or bladder can act like a straightjacket at these organs, causing other problems. These are just a few examples of the pain and/or dysfunctions that adhesions can cause in a variety of bodily systems, including in structures that are in totally different body systems (related only by their proximity to each other), from a fall. Surgeries tend to cause much greater problems, as the body responds to being cut or burned internally.

In General, What Problems Do They Cause?

As seen in the example above, adhesions can cause problems in various parts of the body, areas normally addressed by a variety of medical specialties. The example above caused problems with intercourse and fertility (gynecologic), elimination (urologic), the hip (orthopedic), headaches (neurological) and digestion (gastrointestinal). With such a variety and geography of symptoms, it is no wonder that both the patient and primary physician are confused! Since the original injury happened so long ago, it is long-forgotten. The true cause of the problem, internal adhesions, goes unnoticed because adhesions cannot generally be seen with diagnostic tests.

The challenge in diagnosing the cause of the problem is that adhesions do not appear on tests such as X-rays, CT scans or MRIs. Unable to see them, your physician may send you from specialist to specialist in an attempt to get a definitive diagnosis. Or your doctor may simply say, "There's nothing there." After years of searching for relief, many patients have heard their well-intentioned physician say, "It must all be in your head."

Over the years we have learned that pain and dysfunction that is difficult to diagnose is often caused directly or indirectly by strong, undiagnosed adhesions that formed, often much earlier in life, to help the body heal. Whether from an injury, surgery, infection or endometriosis, adhesive events earlier in life can cause direct and sometimes bizarre, unexplained symptoms and pain patterns in various parts of the body. We will examine the causes of adhesions in more detail in Chapter 2.

How Do I Know If I Have Adhesions?

As you can imagine from the example above, it is nearly impossible to live an active life without developing adhesions. Luckily, we will never notice them in most areas. But when we get unusual or unexplained pain or dysfunction, and physicians are unable to diagnose

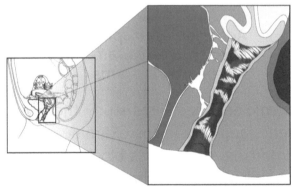

*Adhesions can form after a
bladder or vaginal infection
causing incontinence or significant
intercourse pain, long after the
infection has passed.*

a cause, we should look at healing events earlier in life to determine whether powerful, glue-like adhesions may have formed in areas of the body. When they do, they can bind structures from various bodily systems (digestive, muscular, reproductive, endocrine) that are related geographically by their location in the body, giving mixed, or confusing symptoms.

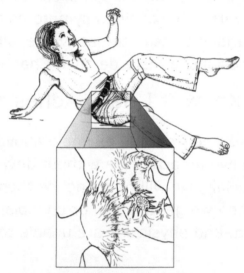

Adhesions can spread to other structures, affecting nearby systems.

In Western medicine, specialists study the body in parts. Medical students and physicians examine bodily systems in various campuses, sometimes blocks or even miles from each other. But the fact that the ovary is located next to the bowel and less than an inch from the inside of the hip, a very active part of our body subject to injury, is not really studied in most medical schools. While orthopedic physicians study the hip, gynecologists study the ovaries, and gastroenterologists study the bowel, none of them have a strong focus on adhesions that can bind structures between bodily systems in a small area, the size of a golf ball. Yet, this geographic proximity is intimately involved in many of the more complex cases we have treated over the last 30 years.

How Big Is The Problem?

Cost in Dollars

The monetary costs of adhesions are astronomical, approaching $50 billion a year! According to the U.S. Department of Human Health Services, adhesion surgery alone costs the U.S. government, insurers and the American public over $11 billion a year. Adhesions are a primary cause of small bowel obstruction, a life-threatening condition in which food can no longer pass through the intestines. Bowel obstruction surgeries cost an additional $16 billion a year. Treating the pain associated with endometriosis, a condition frequently associated with adhesions that bind structures together causing pain or infertility, is over $22 billion a year.

Cost In Human Suffering

As significant as the monetary costs are, they pale in comparison to the cost in human suffering due to adhesions. Many patients with adhesions spend years or decades and thousands of dollars looking for relief – or simply trying to get a diagnosis. During this time, they are sent from doctor to doctor, specialist to specialist. They undergo numerous tests and incredible frustration, only to be told over and over again, "There's nothing there," or "I can't see anything; I'll have to refer you on." Even worse is the inaccurate and rather insulting statement, "It must all be in your head. I'd like to refer you to a psychologist or a psychiatrist."

Indeed, many people start to wonder if they are going crazy due to the difficulties caused by the undiagnosed, unexplained problems that result from adhesions. But, hidden deep within their bodies, these small but powerful structures act like glue, binding internal structures in 'straitjackets' estimated to exert 2,000 pounds a square inch (140 kilos per square centimeter) of pull, while the medical world tells the patient "There's nothing there."

Are Adhesions Different From Scars?

In one sense, adhesions are simply internal scars. This explanation is, perhaps, too simple. External scars are visible and exposed to the outside world. They generally can be seen as a line or, in cases such as burns, as a plane of adhered tissues.

Internally, adhesions can take many forms. They begin in one area as the first step in the process of healing. Then their tendrils may spread to other areas and draw structures together, binding them like internal straitjackets, often decreasing function or causing pain.

Physical Characteristics of Adhesions

What Are They Made of?

Like scars, adhesions are composed of tiny strands of collagen. Like the powerful strands of a nylon rope, these collagen strands form to blanket, surround and isolate areas where tissue has been damaged after a surgery, injury or infection. As they lie down, they bind together in a mass to stop any bleeding that is taking place, and to prevent bacteria that may have entered through damaged skin from spreading to other parts of the body.

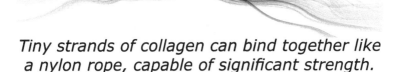

Tiny strands of collagen can bind together like a nylon rope, capable of significant strength.

What Is Their Strength?

The collagen fibers that comprise adhesions have been measured as stronger than steel. Several types of collagen can be found in adhesions but at their very core, the Type 2 collagen fibers that generally form to help the body heal have a tensile strength that has been estimated to approach 2,000 pounds per square inch (140 kilos per square centimeter). If these estimates are even close to correct, you could literally lift a horse with just a small amount of the adhesions that can form within you! Imagine what they are doing to the mobility and functions of your joints, and your delicate organs and nerves.

How Do They Form?

Immediately after a trauma, surgery, infection or inflammation, fibroblasts in the blood stream create thousands of tiny strands of collagen. These strands rush in and lay down on each other in a random pattern to start the process of healing. As they do, a molecular chemical bond attaches each collagen strand to the next and then to the underlying organ, muscle or nerve. Thus, tens of thousands of crosslinks may form as collagen fibers lay down in an area in chaotic patterns.

In general, adhesions continue to form until bleeding and inflammation have stopped and bacteria has been contained. Then, white blood cells and the immune system take over, fighting any infection and continuing the healing process. Once the body has healed, adhesions can remain in the body for a lifetime, as a powerful, permanent but unseen structural bond. Thus, adhesion formation is a natural part of aging throughout life.

What Do They Look Like?

Adhesions can take any number of shapes but, in general, we find that most form within one of the following categories.

Curtains

Filmy adhesions may blanket an area, decreasing sensitivity and the normal elasticity of the tissues. We believe this to be the case when adhesions form on the inner wall of the vagina.

The delicate tissues of this organ have millions of nerve endings designed to elicit pleasure and help the body respond to stimulation. When a vaginal infection occurs – even an undetected subclinical one – adhesions can form on the delicate, nerve-filled walls of the vagina. When

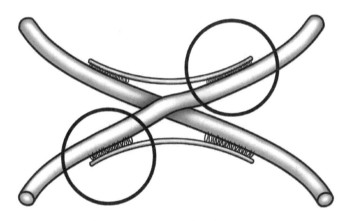

Molecular chemical bonds form between the collagen fibers, and the underlying structures as a first step in adhesion formation.

they do, they can deter normal mobility or block normal sensitivity. Thus arousal, lubrication and orgasm can be adversely affected.

Because these collagen fibers are microscopic and invisible to most diagnostic tests, the physician cannot actually see this curtain in most cases. Thus, the patient is told that "There's nothing there," or "I think it must all be in your head," or simply "Relax and remove some stress from your life." These suggestions are inaccurate and off-putting. Even microscopic collagen bonds can cause significant pain and wreak havoc – in this case, to a woman's love life and relationship. Mechanical problems such as adhesions must be recognized for what they are; then, they can be dealt with mechanically.

Ropes

In some cases, adhesions can form as rope-like structures. In the same way that tiny strands of nylon can create a rope powerful enough to keep a large boat tethered to a dock, adhesions can form together in a rope-like configuration that binds structures together with a powerful force. For example, rope-like adhesions that form after abdominal surgery to help the body heal may spread up to the ribs, pulling the ribcage down toward the public bone.

In this case, it becomes almost impossible to stand up straight as we once did. The patient is pulling against an estimated 2,000 pounds per square inch or more, curling the body forward. The muscles of the upper back and neck begin to hurt as the patient tries to keep the torso from bending further forward, towards the ground.

The patient may think this is a result of age or may be told by a doctor that "There's nothing there; I think you need to start an exercise regimen." But, no amount of exercise can detach the rope-like adhesions that are pulling the patient forward, causing pain in the gut, back, neck or head. For many patients, pain increases after exercise, as they try to pull against these powerful straitjackets.

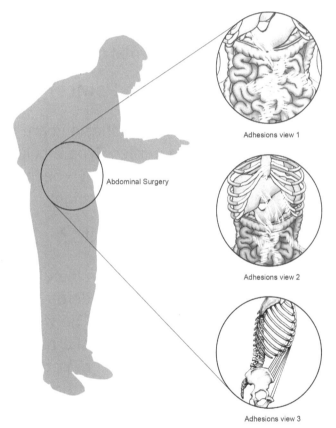

Abdominal Surgery

Adhesions view 1

Adhesions view 2

Adhesions view 3

Adhesions in the abdomen or pelvis can pull the body forward, causing pain in the back or neck as muscles struggle to keep us standing straight.

Balls of String

In some areas, adhesions can resemble a ball or knot of string or rubber bands. We frequently note this occurring in areas of the bowel (intestines) and in large muscle groups such as the glutes (buttocks) or hamstrings. In the upper part of the shoulder, people often notice what are called trigger points. When we palpate these, they feel like balls of string tightly wrapped together. When a manual therapist treats them, pain often decreases as the tissues return to a more normal configuration.

What Are Their Strongest Points?

By far, the strongest elements in adhesions are the collagen fibers. As discussed earlier, Type 2 collagen fibers frequently found in adhesions have been measured to be literally stronger than steel, by weight.

What Are Their Weakest Points?

The good news is that adhesions are vulnerable and apparently capable of deterioration or deformation when their weakest points are manipulated. The weakest points of adhesions are the molecular chemical attachments at which each collagen fiber binds to the next one and the next and, finally, to the underlying structure. Thus, if there is a way to deform or detach or unravel adhesions, we believe that this molecular chemical bond offers our best chance to do that.

Chapter 2
Where Do Adhesions Come From?

Surgery

Surgery is a major cause of adhesion formation in the body – perhaps the most common cause. A massive study of over five decades of surgery published in the journal "Digestive Surgery" showed that 90% of abdominal surgeries and 55% to 100% of pelvic surgeries caused adhesions to form. Ironically, adhesions will form from the very surgeries performed to remove them. Thus, post-surgical adhesions can cause significant problems for surgeons and their patients.

Here's an example: Small bowel obstruction - a life-threatening event in which the intestines become totally blocked (often by adhesions) – will sometimes require surgery to save the patient's life. A 10-year study of over 29,000 patients in the British medical journal "Lancet" showed that over a third (35%) of those who underwent adhesion or bowel obstruction surgery returned to the hospital two or more times over the next 10 years for an adhesion-related hospitalization. In fact, 20% of the patients returned to the hospital within a year, due to problems from adhesions.

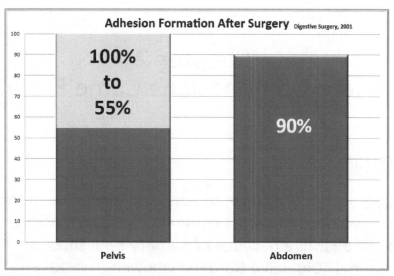

A study of over five decades of post-surgical results adhesions formation highlights the extent of the problem.

Similarly, the U.S. Department of Health and Human Services reported that in 2010, over 18% (about one in five) patients who underwent bowel obstruction surgery returned to the hospital for another surgery within 30 days.

It is clear that while surgery saves lives, a nearly inevitable by-product of surgery is the formation of adhesions. Unfortunately, very few patients are specifically warned of the possibility and consequences of adhesion formation before they undergo surgery. Remarkably, most patients tell us "I was never told about adhesions – why is that?" We will look at this question and possible answers in the next chapter.

Injury and Trauma

Serious injury can cause massive adhesion formation. One of our patients fell asleep in the backseat of a car, only to awaken impaled on the gearshift knob between the front bucket seats when the driver ran into a tree. A child we treated was run over by the twin back wheels of a vehicle, splitting his pelvis open like a book. Both developed massive adhesions from the traumas and the subsequent surgeries to repair their bodies. Both patients nearly lost their lives. Both were facing numerous invasive surgeries to remove adhesions when they decided to learn more about these internal scars. Each of them then took a different, less invasive route, a manual physical therapy to address their adhesions, and regain their lives.

Smaller individual or repetitive traumas also cause adhesions to form as the first step in the healing process. Once the body has healed, adhesions tend to remain in the body, often for the rest of our lives. Some surprising smaller traumas we have seen that caused adhesion formation include:

- A fall while skating;

- A fall off a ladder;

- Years of horseback riding;

- My parents dropped me when I was a child;

- I was in a motor vehicle accident, but didn't develop real pain until a couple years later;

- I was a cheerleader (gymnast, athlete) and I fell on my tailbone (or back, neck, hip, head);

- I performed on uneven parallel bars as a gymnast in school; now as an adult, I have pain (or my fallopian tubes are blocked, or I am infertile), with no apparent explanation;

- Postural trauma such as sitting at the same position, hour upon hour, day after day, year after year with head and shoulders forward (e.g. looking down at schoolwork or a computer monitor);

- Positions at work can require repetitive tasks, such as keeping the arm out to the side for hours at a time. Over time, adhesions form at the inflamed, over-stressed muscles. When they do, they can bind to muscles and nerves, causing pain and/or decreasing normal mobility.

Infection

Any infection can cause adhesions to form. We often see problems after:

- vaginal, blader or yeast infection;

- pelvic inflammatory disease (PID);

- appendicitis;

- post-surgical infection;

- SIBO (small intestine bacterial overgrowth)

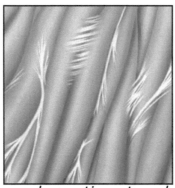

Shown here, tiny strands of collagen can bind individual muscle cells, attaching structures that are designed to move independently.

Inflammation

Conditions that cause inflammation in various parts of the body, for example the liver, stomach or intestines, also result in adhesions. These conditions include:

- endometriosis;

- pancreatitis;

- hepatitis;

- diverticulitis;

- Crohn's disease

Endometriosis

Physicians have not yet identified the exact cause of endometriosis. However, we know that adhesions frequently accompany endometrial implants. We have evidence indicating that as endometrial tissues swell each month, the pull of adhesive fibers called crosslinks is a major cause of the pain associated with endometriosis. Chapter Six provides a more detailed explanation of this process, with a sense of how we can decrease or eliminate the cause of the pain or infertility.

Radiation Therapy

When radiation therapy kills cancer cells, it also destroys nearby cells. We see this often in patients who have undergone cancer treatment, including those with radiation enteritis.

Today, physicians use radiation therapy at much lower intensity than was done in the 1980s and 1990s. Thus, we see more adhesions due to radiation in older patients and those treated under aggressive radiation protocols.

Chapter 3
The Medical Response to Adhesions

How Do Physicians Diagnose Them?

The only definitive way to diagnosis adhesions is through a process called "direct visualization." This means that a physician must perform a surgery in order to see, measure and assess adhesions inside the patient in order to accurately diagnose them. Three challenges facing surgeons are apparent:

1. Surgery generally creates more adhesions.

In order to directly see internal adhesions, the doctor has two choices, both of which are surgical:

i) In a laparoscopy, the physician creates several incisions, then inserts a scope (laparoscope) to view and generally film the adhesions. S/he may cut or burn adhesions that s/he finds.

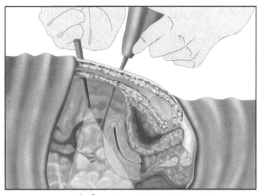

A laparoscopy.

ii) In a laparotomy, the physician creates a larger cut in the skin and underlying muscles or tissues, pulls the sides apart and looks inside to physically view, and remove any visible adhesions.

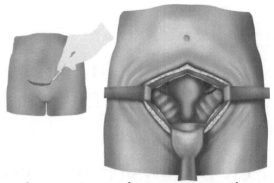

Laparotomy (open surgery).

In both of these situations, the physician gets a direct view of exactly what is happening in the body. However, s/he risks creating more adhesions. While some studies suggest that laparoscopy is less invasive and creates fewer adhesions than laparotomy (open surgery), other studies disagree. One thing is certain – surgery is a primary cause of adhesion formation.

2. Adhesions may be microscopic.

When enough collagen fibers form to make a visible rope, curtain, ball, or any combination of these, the physician can easily diagnose the adhesions. But, as we have learned, the collagen fibers that are the building blocks of adhesions are actually microscopic. Thus, when they form deep within an organ, nerve or other structure, those fibers can cause a significant pull without actually being visible. This can happen wherever they form in the body, causing unexplained pain or problems. As an example, we find this happens deep within the walls of the vagina in cases of decreased sexual function and intercourse pain. Chapter Six addresses these conditions in detail.

3. Adhesions can occur inside of a structure.

The pull of adhesions can cause pain anywhere and can also cause more unusual problems. When crosslinks form between the muscle cells of the hamstring, an athlete cannot run as quickly or stretch his/her leg as far because it is literally adhered by thousands of tiny strands binding cells within the muscle, preventing that leg from stretching out completely.

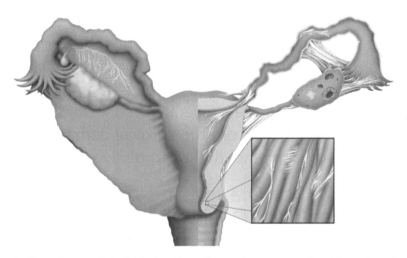

Adhesions (right) in the female reproductive tract.

In the same way, adhesions can and do form between the muscle cells of the cervix or uterus, closing the opening to prevent or deter sperm transfer and creating a much less hospitable surface for embryo implantation.

When these invisible but powerful 'straitjackets' form inside the uterine wall, they can cause spasm or inflammation. This can increase temperature, making implantation difficult and decreasing the opportunity for a fertilized embryo to grow. When they form among cells within the liver or pancreas, they can decrease that organ's function significantly. When they form within the wall of the intestine, they can cause an hourglass shaped restriction called a stricture, creating moderate to severe digestive problems.

Adhesions inside a fallopian tube can completely block that tube, preventing sperm from meeting egg and stopping pregnancy from occurring. While the surgeon can certainly cut into the organs to more directly visualize the adhesions, the damage caused by cutting into these delicate organs – and the subsequent adhesions that form as the body heals from the surgical damage – is generally not recommended if it can be avoided.

Difficulties With Diagnosing Adhesions, or "Why Doesn't My Doctor Believe Me?"

Impossible to See

As we have learned, adhesions are composed of tiny strands of collagen. These fibers lay down in a random pattern to surround and isolate areas of tissue damage in order to start the healing process.

Remarkably, naturally occurring collagen strands cover nearly every structural cell in the body. Virtually every cell that creates a muscle, organ, blood vessel or nerve is surrounded with collagen. Thus, medical equipment manufacturers have been unable to create a diagnostic tool that can distinguish collagenous adhesions from the vast array of structural collagen in the body. X-ray, ultrasound, CT scan or MRI – in most cases, none of these diagnostic tools can show adhesions.

How to Determine the Presence of Adhesions:

1. Direct Visualization

As noted earlier, when a physician can actually see a structure such as an adhesion, this is the most definitive way to diagnose it. Thus, physicians can see adhesions directly through surgery. Unfortunately, as we have seen, surgeries commonly cause more adhesions to form because the body has to heal from the procedure.

2. Indirect Visualization

These include methods such as X-ray, MRI, or CT scan. In an indirect visualization, physicians can often see the effects of adhesions. For example, they may see narrowing at various vessels in the body, such as the intestine or fallopian tube. Using radio opaque dye, they can also see where one structure appears to be pushing or pulling on another.

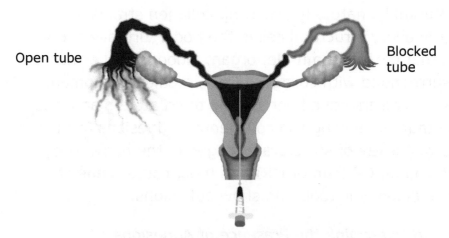

Open tube

Blocked tube

A dye test can indicate likely
adhesion formation, shown here at
the right fallopian tube.

Furthermore, they can see a stricture, the hourglass effect when a hollow vessel narrows in an unexpected area. During a hysterosalpingogram (HSG), physicians may note that dye does not go fully through a fallopian tube or leads a tortuous path on its way to the ovary. Thus, a physician may deduce that adhesions are present without directly visualizing them. The same may be said of other organs, such as the intestine. All of these are examples of indirect visualization, where the diagnostic physician sees the effect but cannot see the adhesion that is causing the problem.

3. History, Symptoms and Palpation

We know that adhesions form as the first step in healing. When the patient reports pain or dysfunction in an area of the body in which an injury, surgery or infection has occurred earlier in life, we can assume that adhesions formed to help the body heal. If the physician has ruled out hormonal or medical causes such as a tumor, we begin to suspect adhesions as the cause of the problem. When a knowledgeable therapist sinks his/her hands into that area, s/he can palpate for hardness, 'ropiness', increased temperature or decreased mobility at, or under the skin. This gives the therapist provider an indirect and non-invasive indication of where adhesions have formed in the body.

Clearly, the more direct methods are more definitive ways of determining that adhesions exist in an area. Just as clearly, the more direct the method, the more invasive the technique for diagnosing, and the greater the chance for creating new adhesions.

Recently, a device called an adheremeter has been scientifically validated as a non-invasive tool for measuring the presence of adhesions. This device was originally designed to assist surgeons to find the safest place to cut the skin, before inserting a laparoscope. The adheremeter is a simple disc with measured concentric circles like a bullseye. When placed on the skin and slid north to south, east to west, and around the clock, it can give a relative diagnosis indicating the extent of adhesions under the skin.

As noted above, the other reasons adhesions are often

difficult to see are that they are invisible to the eye, either because they are:

- microscopic and, thus, too tiny to be recognized, or

- embedded deep within an organ, completely out of sight.

There is no way to see adhesions that are embedded in an organ. These simply cannot be seen without cutting the organ open. This approach risks inflicting significant damage to the organ in order to diagnose adhesions. Naturally, it creates more adhesions in the process, as the body heals from the surgical procedure.

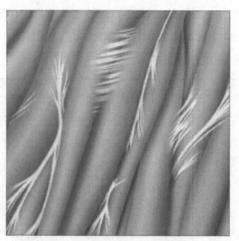

Strong adhesive fiber can
bind cells within a muscle.

In situations where tiny, filmy adhesions form on very delicate tissues, it would be impossible to see them without the use of a microscope. This is not possible in most areas of the body, for example within a muscle or organ, on the vaginal wall or perhaps between the lobes of the liver. In these cases, examining the patient's history of healing events in that area of the body and relating these to his or her symptoms can help determine the likelihood of adhesion formation, without resorting to surgery.

"Adhesions Don't Cause Pain"

Physicians are taught to follow published medical literature. Remarkably, we could find very little medical literature examining specific pain response to adhesions. Part of this may be the fact that adhesions are so difficult to diagnose. Because adhesions can only be directly diagnosed through surgery (when the patient cannot feel pain), a physician cannot diagnose pain when a patient is under general anesthesia. Thus, many doctors focus on relieving pain with analgesics (painkillers).

Medicine has become very specialized in the last few decades. Most specialties do not include a study of adhesions other than recognizing that they can form after surgery and that anything that prevents their formation would benefit the patient. Those who do specialize in treating adhesions are generally surgeons who naturally want to directly visualize them; then they will cut or burn the adhesions under general anesthesia in order to relieve the patient's pain, or improve function.

While so many physicians are brilliant, compassionate and highly accomplished professionals, most medical schools do not appear to equip them with a thorough understanding of the steps involved in adhesive bonding. None that we know of have ever found ways to deform or dissolve those bonds non-surgically. Instead, they turn to scalpels or lasers to cut or burn through the adhesions.

Let Me Refer You On

Unable to see the adhesions that are causing their patients problems, many physicians come to the conclusion that "This condition is out of my domain; I need to refer you on." Thus, many patients with chronic adhesion pain or dysfunction are referred from specialist to specialist in an attempt to diagnose the condition. Assuming the problem is finally diagnosed as adhesion-related, the patient's options are to live with the condition until it becomes unbearable or undergo a surgery to cut or burn the adhesions, and remove what they can.

Maybe It's All in Your Head

At some point, many patients we treat for adhesion pain or dysfunction have been told, "It's all in your head; let me refer you to a psychiatrist or a psychologist." Having spent years searching for the cause of their pain and obtaining no answer from specialist after specialist, yet profoundly affected by these bonds that are causing chronic or recurring pain, being told that "It's all in your head" is incredibly disempowering for the patient.

Understand that the physicians are not trying to belittle you or your concerns; they just do not have an answer for you. They cannot see the problem or feel it and it does not appear on any diagnostic tests. Rather than telling you "I don't know what this is," some physicians conclude "It must all be in your head."

Know this – if you are feeling pain in your body, there is a cause. It is real and it is usually exactly where you are feeling it. If your physician has been unable to find it, if there is no disease and no medical or hormonal reason for it, and if nothing definitive appears on diagnostic tests, it is reasonable to assume that you have adhesions.

Looking at Your Life History

Adhesions form as the body's first step in healing. To begin determining whether adhesions are causing your problem, it is necessary to review your lifetime history for falls, injuries, infections and surgeries dating back to birth. Think about what happened in or near your problem area a few years before you began having pain or dysfunction. If you recall something, you may have your first hint of the underlying cause of your pain or dysfunction.

Look back at your history; notice where you are hurting. Is there something in your history that occurred near the part of your body where your pain or dysfunction is occurring? If so, when did that take place? If adhesions are the cause, these events will often have happened one to three years before the pain starts.

In some cases, healing events that cause adhesions may have occurred decades earlier. Quite a few of the patients we have treated over the years underwent surgery at birth. When this happens, the surgery creates scarring and the child has to grow around the scar. In general, scars do not often dissipate as we grow. Instead, the body tends to grow around an adhered area, leading to pain or dysfunction years, or even decades later in life.

We suggest you try the following: lay back and relax, then let your hands sink in at either side of your abdomen or pelvis. Now, slowly bring your hands together, gathering the tissues between them. This gentle compression allows spasm and increased tone of the muscles to relax.

Now, remove your hands and let your fingers sink in at various areas, including areas where you feel pain or discomfort. You may want to compare left versus right side. Do your hands sink in like they are sinking into soft, supple tissue or is there resistance? Do your fingers ever run into something that feels hard, perhaps the texture of broccoli under your skin or some 'ropiness' that causes you discomfort – perhaps on one side of your body more than the other? If so, this is a sign that you likely have adhesions in that area. You can try the same experiment anywhere you have pain.

Doctors Ignore Patient Complaints of Pain

Pain Is Natural (Especially in Women)

Even in the 21st century, some health care providers continue to feel that all women have some degree of pain and that this is natural. While pain may be natural, it is not a good thing. Pain indicates that something is wrong. If you are feeling pain, there is a reason for it. Statements such as "Everyone has some pain" or "It is natural for women to have pain" are inaccurate and misleading. If there is pain, there is a problem and there is a cause for the pain.

Diagnosis: Need Second Opinions/Specialist

Most people with longstanding pain have been referred to other specialist physicians. Examples include being referred to an orthopedic surgeon, a neurologist for testing, a gastroenterologist for bowel issues, a gynecologist for female complaints, a physiatrist for a musculoskeletal diagnosis or a psychiatrist for the "all in your head" diagnosis. If you find yourself on this merry-go-round, consider the possibility that you have adhesions – a mechanical problem invisible to generalists and most specialists, rather than a disease-related or hormonal condition.

What Can My Doctor Do About Adhesions?

If your doctor feels that you have adhesions the medical response is going to generally follow this tract:

1) "There is nothing to do about adhesions except surgery. If the adhesions are bad enough and are severely interrupting your life, I can perform a surgery to cut or burn the adhesions I can find."

Your doctor may or may not tell you that surgery will create more adhesions. Know that s/he is not trying to be deceptive. No matter how skilled the physician, all surgeries tend to create more adhesions as the body's delicate tissues heal from being cut or burned.

Some physicians feel that there is no sense in telling patients about adhesions and worrying them, since post-surgical adhesion formation is nearly inevitable.

2) Your physician may prescribe pain medications or refer you to a pain specialist, generally an anesthesiologist. That physician may suggest a nerve block or injections such as steroids into the adhered area to decrease the pain and inflammation.

Pain-relieving medications and nerve blocks do not change anything physically in the structure of your body, or address the adhesions. They simply mask the pain.

If you choose to undergo surgery, you may have great

relief that lasts for years or a lifetime. Some patients get relief for a period of time but once post-surgical adhesions form, the pain returns sometimes worse than before. Some patients report that surgery did not help them at all or made things worse. In all of these cases, the doctor is making structural changes in your body to decrease the adhesions. As noted above, the problem is that new adhesions tend to form to help you heal.

Various gels and surgical meshes have been tried to decrease surgical adhesion formation. We suggest you speak with your doctor about his or her experience with these. Clinically, we have not seen significant success with any of those approaches. When meshes are introduced, they can become another substance to which new adhesions bind.

Surgery: Causes More Adhesions to Form

Surgery is your doctor's only option for directly visualizing the adhesions. The advantage is that they do get to see exactly what is going on, and that they can then cut or burn adhesions. A primary disadvantage is possible formation of new adhesions. Other risks include "inadvertent enterotomy," when a physician mistakenly cuts or damages a nearby organ. This can happen when adhesions are so thick that the surgeon cannot see through them, or if a hand or instrument slips during a surgery.

If that physician happens to cut any of the 21 feet (7

meters) of the small intestines and a bit of intestinal contents leak out, the patient often develops a serious internal infection. In that case, the surgeon must perform a repeat surgery, administer antibiotics directly to the site of the inadvertent cut, stitch the area up again, and perhaps leave the wound open to heal from the inside out. In this case, the patient develops extensive adhesions due to the two successive surgeries, on both sides of a serious internal infection.

A recent risk now being explored is the risk to the brain from recurring use of the anesthesia administered during surgery. Thus, if your surgeon is reluctant to perform surgery to see what is going on, you now understand why. There are significant risks associated with opening your body to perform a surgery, beyond the formation of additional adhesions.

Is There Anything Natural I Can Do To Decrease My Adhesions?

Recent data shows that there may be other options for people who have adhesions. Studies in medical journals are indicating that a type of manual physical therapy can and does decrease adhesions. Published studies on recurring adhesive conditions are promising. We will touch on those in the last chapter of this book.

Chapter 4
Adhesions and Chronic Pain

Background

After relieving Belinda of the severe pelvic pain she experienced after surgery and radiation therapy, she and her husband opened a small clinic specializing in the treatment of chronic pain caused by adhesions. They felt that other people like her suffered from adhesion pain that was difficult or impossible to diagnose without surgery. They suggested doctors in their area refer patients with chronic unexplained pain – the ones they could not fix. They were surprised to find that physicians filled their schedule quickly, referring scores of patients with unexplained pain within the first few weeks. Many of these had unusual or complex pain patterns, some dating back many years or even decades. Yet when the therapists compared the patient's areas of pain or dysfunction with areas of prior injury, infection, surgery or endometriosis, they began to see strong parallels.

Overview

Many patients spend years or decades searching for relief from chronic, often unexplained pain. Their physicians order test after test to determine the cause of the pain – yet none of the tests show anything. The tests are deemed "inconclusive."

"How can it be that nothing shows up?" the patient asks. "I know I have pain. I can feel it very specifically, right here."

It's not that your physician is not skilled; the problem is the difficulty diagnosing adhesions. Medical science is highly equipped to test for medical, hormonal and organic conditions such as diseases, chemical imbalances or erratic markers in the blood. But except for the adheremeter (which can test for superficial adhesions, those near the skin), there are no definitive tests for adhesions and the powerful internal scars that form wherever in our body heals. Thus, your physician may be looking for organic, medical or hormonal causes for your pain when the cause is actually mechanical.

Causes of Mechanical Problems Can Be Difficult To Diagnose

A variety of noninvasive tests can diagnosis some mechanical dysfunctions. From the least expensive X-rays to sophisticated MRIs, CT scans and PET scans, diagnostic tests can note subluxations, asymmetries, and problems in joints and many organs of our body. Once diagnosed, the questions become 1) What is causing the mechanical problem? and 2) What can we do about it?

Most patients with chronic pain have tried a variety of massage or chiropractic techniques to treat their pain. Many people note relief from those treatments; the problem is that relief does not last. The pain returns.

If massage or chiropractic care have provided you with some relief, it is a good indication that your chronic pain is likely mechanical in nature. Rather than a disease or hormonal condition that may be treated with drugs, some of the structural elements of your body have become pulled out of their usual orientation, causing pain or dysfunction.

Adhesions are powerful mechanical bonds that form in the body as the first step in the healing process. After the body has healed, adhesions can remain in the body for a lifetime. Pound for pound, adhesions have been measured as stronger than steel. As they spread, they can squeeze, pull on or bind together structures that should be free to move independently. Below, we will look at some of the chronic conditions caused by adhesions. If you have any of these and the diagnosis has been elusive, adhesions from an earlier healing event may be the cause of your pain.

Pain After Surgery

As we saw in Chapter Two, surgery is a major cause of internal adhesions. In fact, surgery is frequently cited as the primary cause of recurring bowel obstruction, a life-threatening condition in which the intestines are squeezed shut by adhesions. Unable to eat, the patient will die in 100% of cases unless the obstruction clears via surgery, therapy or on its own.

The epidermis (skin) is designed to keep the outside

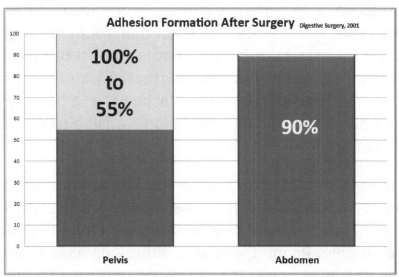

A 50+ year study of Western medical literature found adhesions formed after 55% to 100% of abdominal and pelvic surgeries. Digestive surgery 2001

world from intruding on the inner spaces of our body. When our skin is cut or scraped, fibroblasts exude tiny collagen fibers to create a scar as quickly as possible in order to keep the inner workings of our body safe from intrusion by bacteria from the outside world.

Thus, when a surgeon cuts deeply into our body to enter the innermost sanctums of our muscles, organs and nerves, s/he does so with a significant amount of preparation and caution.

Unfortunately, no matter how brilliant and skilled the physician, the cutting and burning of live tissue deep inside of the body always elicits a deep healing response. In order to start the recovery process, fibroblasts in the body creates thousands of tiny collagen strands. These strands rush in to blanket the area that has been cut, burned or damaged by the surgery and to create an internal scar – an adhesion to start the healing process.

Ideally, the internal scar forms exactly at the site where the patient has been cut or burned, without spreading to other areas. In this case, the body creates a neat repair in exactly the spot where it is needed, without creating glue-like bonds that attach to other structures.

But in many cases, adhesions tend to also form in nearby areas that were damaged or inflamed, spreading from structure to structure and from nerve to nerve, binding them in a powerful internal 'straitjacket'. Muscles, organs, ligaments and nerves, any or all of these structures can become entwined in these strong internal bonds.

In a scenario we frequently see, the patient returns to work. Sitting in a chair, looking at a computer monitor month after month, year after year, adhesions can spread in the forward-flexed body, binding structures along the chest, or the front of the abdomen or pelvis.

A year or two later, the patient begins to notice pain in the abdomen, back, neck or along her side, and wonders where it is coming from. She goes to the doctor for a diagnosis but nothing is found. "There's nothing there," the physician says. "At least I can't see anything. Let me refer you to a specialist for some tests."

Thus the patient begins a search for an answer to the adhesions that have formed during the months or years after surgery, that are now causing pain. The problem is not that the surgeon did something wrong; it is simply a result of the body's pattern of healing from surgery.

Where and how adhesions form geographically within the body varies greatly. Many people have no problems or symptoms at all after surgery. But for some, the adhesions that initially formed to help the body heal from surgery continue to spread for months, years or decades, causing pain later in life.

Back and Hip Pain

Back pain has plagued humankind for centuries. Finding the cause of back pain and its cure can be a daunting, sometimes elusive, undertaking. Because the sacrum, pelvis and lower back are transition points between the legs (lower body) and the torso (upper body), back pain is often caused by a mechanical problem that originates in the joints and connective tissues of these transition areas. Mechanical problems can and should be treated mechanically, starting with the safest, most conservative approach. This approach follows the physician's Hippocratic Oath, "above all, do no harm." This is often translated as "prescribe therapy before drugs, and drugs before surgery."

Back, hip or tailbone injuries can cause both direct and indirect trauma to the back. Accidents or injuries that affect transitional areas can create adhesions as the first step in the healing process. Tailbone injuries can pull down on the dura, the collagenous sleeve that envelopes the spinal cord, compressing some of the nerve roots of the spine. In these cases, the adhesions that formed to help us heal can become our nemesis. They may grow over time and create a constant pulling force in our back, hip, tailbone, or the base of our skull causing intermittent or constant pain in those or nearby areas.

Traumas or surgeries at the abdomen can also cause back problems. Adhesions that form after a surgery in the abdomen or pelvis can attach to the front of the vertebrae in our lower back. Over time, they can pull those vertebrae forward, causing a subluxation or misalignment that causes pain by creating a constant or intermittent pull on these vertebrae, the spinal cord and the nerve roots they enclose, even with the smallest movement.

The same adhesive mechanism can affect women with endometriosis. Adhesions that form around endometrial implants tend to create internal straitjackets that pull on structures where endometrial implants form, in the abdomen, back, hip, coccyx or reproductive structures, resulting in pain.

Chronic Migraines, Headaches

The human body was not designed to sit at a desk, with our torso flexed forward and our head tilted back so we could see our school books or computer monitor. Nor were we designed to have a telephone headset lifted by our shoulder to our ear or our hand extended on our computer mouse for hours at a time. Our bodies were designed to wander and move freely while hunting and gathering, varying our postures widely during the course of the day.

When we sit at a desk for hours at a time, month after month, year after year, our bodies develop chronic postures that can create unusual pulls at the base of our skull and into our head.

Most of the chronic pain patients we have seen over the last 30 years have also complained of

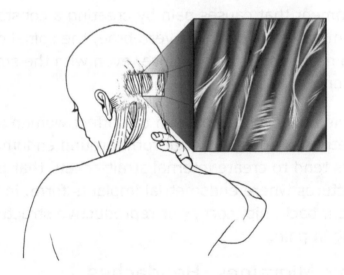

We find adhesive tissue at the base of the skull is common in people with recurring headaches.

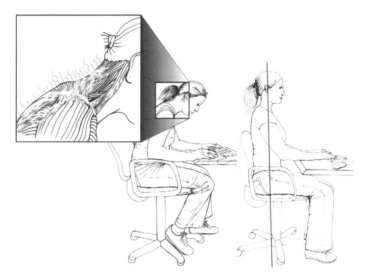

*Our sitting positions can cause chronic
neck pain or headaches, later in life.*

headaches. For the great majority of these, treating
adhered tissues, starting at the pelvis and back, then
moving up through the neck, and finally treating the soft
tissues at the base of the skull has been the missing link
that unlocks those headaches. The same can be said of
our patients with other migraine symptoms such as visual
or auditory sensitivity, nausea or light headedness.

Looking at a sitting or standing body from the side,
one should be able to draw a vertical line through the
ear, through the shoulder and hip joints, and straight
down to the ground. But when our bodies are flexed
forward, the muscles in our upper back and neck must
work constantly in order to keep our heads from falling
forward. At the same time, the muscles at the top of our
neck work twice as hard to keep our head extended back
so that we can see our computer monitors. Due to these

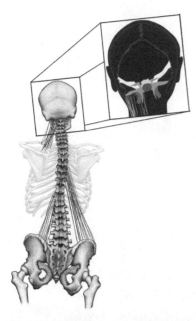

Adhesions can create whole body problems.

muscles working overtime, the pulls at the base of our skull can become significant sources of pain at the upper back, neck or head.

Hoping to help muscles that go into spasm after hours of fixed posture, the body sends in collagenous crosslinks, the building blocks of adhesions, to assist the muscles of the back and neck. As these crosslinks lay down, they bind together muscle cells that are designed to work independently. This can create a thickened, rope-like texture at muscles that should be supple. In short, the soft tissues begin to be bound in adhesions.

The cranium is comprised of 22 major bones, not including the teeth. These bones actually have tiny joints between them, allowing the head to expand and contract about eight times a minute. In doing this, the cranium pumps cerebrospinal fluid down to the tailbone and back up again, lubricating the spinal cord through a covering called the dura. When adhered structures below the head pull down on the delicate bones that comprise the skull, the cranial bones can be pulled out of their normal anatomical alignment. This not only interrupts the pumping mechanism that lubricates the spinal cord, it can cause a host of other problems.

There are millions of nerves at the base of the skull and within the cranium. The brain and structures within the cranium control many of our bodily functions including vision, balance, and hormones, as well as sensations such as pain. When powerful adhesive bonds pull on the delicate cranial structures, they can cause a variety of symptoms from blurred vision and imbalance to significant pain.

Because diagnostic tests for patients with migraines or headaches generally do not assess adhesions, patients may be given pain relievers or nerve blocks. These "treatments" temporarily mask the pain without addressing its root cause. Thus, many still go to the emergency room regularly for pain relief. Once the mechanical malalignments and adhesions are addressed, we find that symptoms generally ease or completely resolve.

TMJ/TMD

The jaw joint is also called the tempero-mandibular joint (TMJ). It is named for the two bones that connect there – the temporal bone, which contains the ear canal and your center of balance, and the mandible, the jaw that holds your lower teeth. Problems at the TMJ are often referred to as tempero-mandibular dysfunction, or TMD.

The TMJ is a bilateral joint, which means that it exists on both sides of the body at the same time. As a very mobile joint used with every bite we take and every word we speak, the TMJ gets a tremendous amount of use.

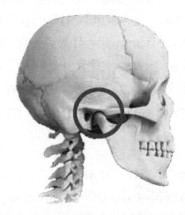

Due to its placement above the spinal cord, this joint is subject to imbalances that occur in all of the structures below, including the feet, legs, pelvis, spine and neck. Thus, many dentists and their patients find that equilibrating teeth (filing down or building up) to help align the TM joint may be ineffective and counterproductive unless asymmetries in the larger support structures of the legs, pelvis, back and neck are treated first.

Clinically, we have found that traumas, surgeries and chronic poor posture over time can create adhesive responses, pulling structural elements of the body below the TMJ out of their natural symmetry. Any malalignment from the feet to the base of the skull can affect this bilateral joint at the top of the body, a joint that rests on virtually everything below it. Thus, an effective protocol to address tempero-mandibular dysfunction (TMD) involves first stepping back and assessing the symmetry of the entire body. Are the hips and pelvis level? Are the shoulders and neck symmetrical, or are they being pulled out of alignment? Is there a scoliosis in the back? If so, how do these malalignments affect the jaw?

It makes sense to first work to correct the large support elements below the TMJ, rather than going immediately into the mouth to equilibrate by filing down or building up the teeth.

If we start by adjusting the teeth, what happens to the jaw alignment if the patient later has bodywork to align the rest of the body? This simply begins a new series of structural problems at the TM joint.

As noted earlier, the strength of adhesions can surpass steel. Thus, adhered tissues pulling structures below the TM joint out of alignment can adversely affect the balance of this delicate bilateral joint. Grinding the teeth down or building them up is like putting a Band Aid on a broken bone. Unless any malalignment, from the feet to the neck is addressed first, dental equilibration is a temporary solution that does not address the core of the problem. It is necessary to first address the adhesions that are pulling body out of alignment. Then, the dentist can look at what s/he calls the "vertical dimension" within the TM joint and make any necessary adjustments *after* the adhesions have been decreased and symmetry has returned to the body.

> *Night Guards for Teeth Grinding: Grinding the teeth and clinching during sleep is a common source of TMJ pain. Many doctors will recommend the use of a night guard to stop damage to the condyles, which are the small shock absorbers between the mandible and temporal bones. While we find night guards can be useful, we strongly recommend the use of a lower rather than an upper night guard to decrease the pain that comes from nighttime clinching, called bruxing. A lower night guard rests on the teeth and grasps only one bone, the mandible (jaw). An upper splint will lock the twin bones of the left and right maxillae (cheek bones) together. If the bones of the cranium are already out of alignment, an upper splint that binds the misaligned maxillae will tend to reinforce that asymmetry, perpetuating the problem.*

Adhesion-Related Disorder (ARD)

When adhesions become so extensive that they affect multiple areas of the body, this condition may be called adhesion-related disorder, or ARD. Patients with ARD may not benefit from surgery. They already have extensive adhesions and, as we have seen, surgery tends to create more adhesions.

Medications can help mask the pain. Most people we see with ARD have been suffering for years or decades, and they simply want their lives back. In order to decrease the pain, it is necessary to address the adhesive tissues wherever they exist within the body.

All physicians in the U.S. take an oath to follow the creed "Above all, do not harm." This generally translates to start treatment with the most conservative approach first. With ARD, we find that following that creed means to try therapy before medications, drugs before surgery, and surgery as a last resort.

Chapter 5
Life-Threatening Intestinal Adhesions

Bowel Obstructions: When Adhesions Become Life Threatening

It is remarkable to think that something that is composed of tiny microscopic strands and is invisible to nearly all modern diagnostic tests can be so painful and debilitating – and even kill you. But that is exactly the case when adhesions form in and around the loops of the small intestines – the bowel.

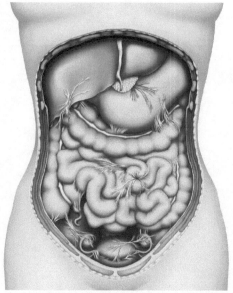

Adhesions in the bowel can be dangerous or life-threatening.

Adults have roughly 21 feet (7 meters) of intestines. As the organ that is primarily concerned with our nutrition, this long, sinuous tunnel runs back and forth, up and down between our stomach and throughout our abdomen, finally turning into our large intestine at the right lower quadrant of the torso.

For most people, the bowel functions well throughout life. But when the abdomen or pelvis has undergone surgery (e.g. C-section, hysterectomy, tummy tuck, endometriosis, lysis of adhesions), an infection (e.g.

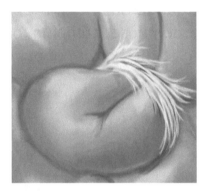

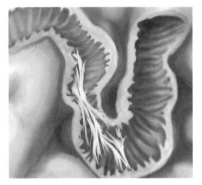
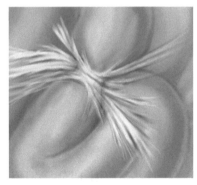

Various types of bowel obstruction.

Crohns, colitis, diverticulitis, a burst appendix, or a severe injury, can cause adhesions to form, to help the body heal. As shown in the images on the previous page, they can create straitjackets among the loops of the intestines.

If adhesions merely form on the outside of the bowel and do not squeeze them, symptoms can be minimal or non-existent. Adhesions become a problem when they decrease the intestines' motility, the movement that pushes food through the bowel to the large intestine. Adhesions become dangerous when they squeeze or kink the bowel like a garden hose, stopping food from moving through and exiting at the bottom of our digestive tract.

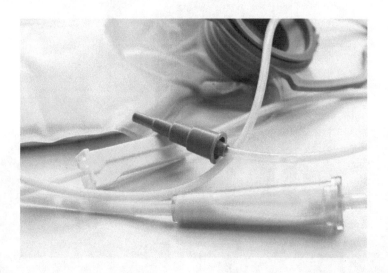

Life-threatening problems occur when adhesions partially or totally block the intestines. Food cannot go through; it backs up. The patient first becomes nauseous, then experiences pain that has been described as beyond excruciating.

The patient is rushed to the hospital emergency room where an NG (nasogastric) tube may be inserted through the nose, down the esophagus and into the stomach. The attendant will attach a pump to the far end and pump out the stomach contents to relieve pressure on the digestive system. The patient quickly receives intravenous needles to allow the hospital team to hydrate the body with saline, to provide liquid nutrition (because the body can no longer ingest food), and to inject strong opiate-based pain relievers. The patient may undergo a CT scan so that physicians can see exactly where the blockage is occurring. While they will not be able to see the adhesions, they may be able to see the blockage that the adhesions are causing or note swelling of the bowel just above the blockage.

Having done all of this, the physician tells the patient "Now, we just have to wait."

The patient says, "What do you mean, we just have to wait? Can't we do something?"

"No, there's really nothing to be done but wait to see if it clears. If it does, you will be able to go home. Nothing will have changed structurally and this may occur again in fact, that is likely. But at least you will have dodged a bullet this time," the doctor says.

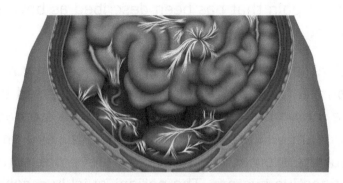

Surgery often creates adhesions.

The average hospital stay for bowel resection surgery is 14.2 days, according to the U.S. Department of Health and Human Services and the average cost is $114,175. Thus, patients lie in bed with IV tubes as their only source of nutrition for an average of two weeks, hoping the obstruction clears. This entire time, patients have an NG tube running through their esophagus, throat and nose, pumping out their stomach. Generally, the only thing they are allowed to have in their mouth is ice. Finally, the physician says, "We're going to have to operate if the obstruction has not passed."

"What is that like?" asks the patient.

"We'll make a small cut to start; hopefully, I can treat you with a laparoscopy, which is less invasive. If you are too adhered, we're going to have to transition to a full open surgery."

Some surgeons pull out all 21 feet of the small intestine, inspecting it inch-by-inch for adhesions, lesions or problems. If they see blockages, strictures (narrowing) or necrotic (dead) tissue, they cut out the problem sections, then re-attach the good parts that remain.

"What about afterwards?" the patient asks. "What's my life going to be like afterwards?"

"You will almost certainly have to adapt to a compromised diet; 18% of patients return to the hospital within 30 days for another hospitalization (according to the U.S. Department of Health and Human Services). Part of the problem is that there is a chance of bowel contents containing bacteria leaking into the interstitial spaces of the body (between the loops of the bowel). This can cause a serious infection. In that case, we will have to quickly perform another surgery to treat the infection. We will do our best to prevent that from happening during surgery, but even a drop or two of bowel contents leaking out where we cut can cause this to occur."

"Unfortunately, there's nothing that we can do to prevent you from having future bowel obstructions. If adhesions form at the site where we've cut or anywhere in the intestines, they can re-occlude (close again) the bowel, possibly creating another obstruction and the need for another surgery." In fact, 35% of patients who undergo bowel obstruction surgery are rehospitalized due to adhesions, 22% in the first year after surgery, per a large study in *Lancet*.

For some patients, the problems related to bowel

obstruction end after an initial surgery. But for more than a third of patients, that surgery marks the beginning of a series of serious adhesive or digestive problems and surgeries that continue throughout their lives.

Other than death, perhaps the worst of these episodes are the recurring "partial bowel obstructions" that take place after an initial surgery. We have treated many patients who have had three, four or more successive surgeries for adhesions and bowel obstructions. These patients often feel stuck in a vicious cycle of adhesions, pain, obstruction, and surgery, with no end in sight.

Surgeons and physicians are generally highly skilled, compassionate professionals but despite the greatest skills, no surgeon can prevent adhesions from forming. Doctors do their best to create barriers for adhesion formation using films and gels, but many surgeons find that these are far less effective than they would like. Sometimes, the mesh used to prevent adhesions ends up caught within a web of adhesions that then needs to be removed, along with the new adhesions that attach it to the existing structures.

Decreased Motility

Motility refers to the natural movement of each organ within itself. In the intestines, this largely refers to peristalsis, the pushing of food down the digestive tract. Adhesive bonds that decrease this natural movement of food through the digestive tract can cause recurring constipation, pain, bloating and even diarrhea. If the adhesions cause a kink in the intestine or squeeze it shut, they may lead to one or more adhesive bowel obstructions.

Small Intestinal Bacterial Overgrowth (SIBO)

SIBO is defined as the proliferation of bacteria that are normally found in the large intestines up in the small intestines. These bacteria do not belong in the small intestine in any significant number. When they appear there, they can cause a variety of symptoms, including constipation, diarrhea, bloating, inflammation, pain and serious weight loss. In fact, the bacteria characteristic of SIBO can eat the food we consume, preventing us from getting adequate nutrition. This is a very serious condition. Treatment may involve low dose antibiotics, given over several weeks. Adhesions appear to decrease the effectiveness of these medications, such that the symptoms return time and again.

Saving a Life: SIBO and Adhesions

A physician said that her patient with SIBO was not responding to treatment medications. The patient's weight was down to 86 pounds and she was getting iron infusions regularly. Her BMI of 16 was categorized as "severely underweight." She was so weak that she arrived at our clinic in a wheelchair.

After we treated her adhesions, the medications began working. She regained her normal weight and had no further need for a wheelchair. In concert with several physicians, we deduced that adhesions in her intestines were preventing the treated bacteria from leaving her body. Once we were able to decrease or eliminate the adhesions, the treated bacteria could exit her body, preventing a re-proliferation of SIBO bacteria and allowing her to return to her normal life.

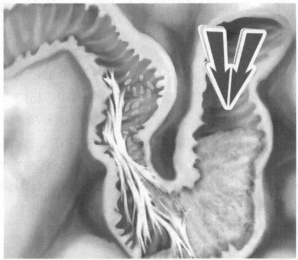

Bowel adhesions can prevent treated
bacteria from leaving the body.

SIBO is common in patients who have undergone prior bowel, pelvic or abdominal surgery. This is especially true for those who have had their ileo-cecal valve removed. This is the valve between the small and large intestines. When it is intact, it tends to prevent bacteria from traveling up into the small intestines. But after a surgeon removes it, as frequently happens in bowel surgery, bacteria from the large intestines are free to matriculate up into the small intestine, creating a fertile environment for SIBO bacteria to proliferate.

SIBO also tends to occur in people who have undergone a significant food poisoning event. In some cases, the inflammation from the unintended bacterial activity in the small intestines creates adhesions, which further slow or prevent the exit of treated bacteria from the body. For many people this creates a cycle of bacteria, adhesions, treatment, proliferation of the remaining bacteria, followed by more inflammation and more adhesions. Decreasing or eliminating adhesions tends to break that cycle, as the treated bacteria can now exit the body.

Digestive Disorders (IBS, Ulcerative Colitis, Crohn's)

Digestive diseases such as the ones noted above are not directly caused by adhesions. However, because adhesions form due to inflammation or infection, these conditions can cause or perpetuate adhesions. Physicians often have difficulty treating these conditions, which tend to recur over a person's life.

When adhesive straitjackets form at tissues that have been inflamed by irritable bowel syndrome (IBS), colitis or Crohn's, it may be difficult to tell whether the condition itself or the resulting adhesions are the cause of the pain and digestive symptoms. In chronic cases, it is likely a combination of both. Coupled with dietary modifications and medications, a conservative therapy to decrease adhesions without surgery may benefit these patients. If an active infection exists or a flare of Crohn's symptoms we find that manual therapy generally should not be applied until the infection or flare have been treated.

CHAPTER 6
Adhesions and Women's Health

Stopping Fertility, Causing Pain, Making Sex Unbearable

Overview

Women are especially susceptible to adhesions for several reasons. These include their unique anatomy, external environment, internal environment and the delicacy and complexity of their pelvic organs. Women are often the medical caretakers for the family, a fact that may cause them to undergo more exploratory surgeries than men, as they try to determine the cause of their pain or dysfunction.

Falls on the Tailbone

All of us – men, women and children – are subject to

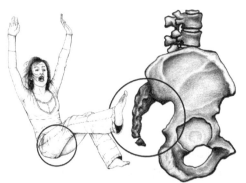

Falls onto the coccyx are common occurances.

injury to our tailbone (coccyx) from early in life. A fall onto the tailbone while running, skating or playing is common in most medical histories.

When this occurs, the ligaments that hold our tailbone in position, like the ropes that hold a tent pole, may be injured and shortened. When collagen crosslinks lay down to help start the healing process from a fall onto our bottom, they generally form at the ligaments on one or both sides of the tailbone. This can pull the coccyx forward and prevent it from extending back as it normally does in life, when needed.

Even much later in life, that forward pull on the tailbone can cause constipation or difficulty sitting for long periods of time. Having in a sense "closed the door" at our bottom, the forward tailbone can make bowel movements

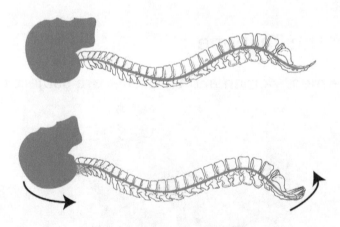

A forward tailbone can often create a
strong pull at the base of the skull.

become more difficult. The result can contribute to constipation, painful, strained bowel movements or other problems.

Among other things, this forward position can create a strong pull on the dura, which surrounds the spinal cord all the way to attachments at the base of the skull and into the head. In fact, we have found the pull of a forward tailbone to be linked to headaches that start at the top of the neck and the base of the skull. When the tailbone is pushed forward a half-inch or a centimeter,

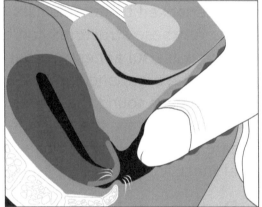

When it feels like your partner is hitting something, he generally is, usually we find it is a forward coccyx or an adhered cervix.

it pulls the covering of the spinal cord down. This can cause pain in the lower back or at the base of the skull, precipitating back pain or headaches. Additionally, this adhesive pull from a fall onto one's bottom can cause prostate problems for some men, leading to pain with ejaculation, erection, orgasm or bowel movements.

For women, a fall on the tailbone can have significant, sometimes severe consequences. A fall onto the coccyx can elicit pain with deep intercourse (dyspareunia); her partner is literally striking the coccyx and its tightened ligaments during sex. As we will see, adhesions in this area can also cause or contribute to female infertility. These subjects are covered more thoroughly later in this chapter.

For patients seeking relief from pelvic pain, infertility or chronic headaches, the tailbone can be a very important area that can be overlooked by neurologists, urologists and gynecologists. Yet these structures can be profoundly affected by the tiny, powerful adhesions that form after any healing event in the area, and can last a lifetime. In a very real sense, we have found that pelvic adhesions that formed at an early age are the "missing link" for many women searching for relief from pain, infertility or decreased sexual function.

Destroying Dreams of Motherhood

Blocked Fallopian Tubes

Background: After receiving soft tissue treatment for adhesions, our female patient was surprised that both of her fallopian tubes opened and she became pregnant. She had been intimate with the same partner for seven years; she said that she never used contraceptives because she didn't need to. Early diagnostic tests showed that both of her fallopian tubes were totally blocked.

Surprised to see that her tubes opened after therapy, and knowing that adhesions are a primary cause of tubal occlusion (blockage), we began to research whether it is possible to treat female infertility by addressing adhesions. We have since published several studies on this phenomenon with positive results, the latest being a 10-year study of nearly 1,400 infertile women.

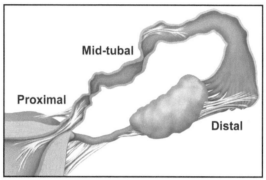

Adhesions can form anywhere in the fallopian tube.

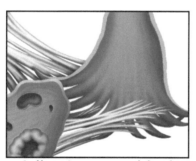

Adhesions can block the end of the fallopian tube, by the ovary.

We first learned of the effect of adhesions on female fertility when treating patients with chronic pelvic pain. Several patients, including a referring physician's wife, became pregnant despite years of totally blocked fallopian tubes. Radiologic tests conducted before and after therapy showed that blocked tubes opened in her, and several other women. Most of those whose tubes opened went on to become pregnant naturally, showing both structural and functional improvements.

Adhesions form to help the body heal from infection and inflammation. After healing, they remain in the body, blocking the fallopian tubes. Thus, the sperm never has a chance to enter the tube to meet the egg, so conception cannot occur. Fallopian tubes can become blocked for several reasons, but tubal occlusion is generally considered a mechanical condition. Pelvic inflammatory disease tends to block fallopian tubes proximally – near the uterus.

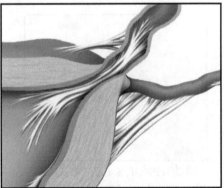

Proximal occlusion occurs where the tube exits the uterus.

Women with prior hip injuries, appendicitis, surgery or endometriosis would often present with blockage at the far end of the tube (distally), next to the ovary.

Looking more closely at the anatomy, we note that the inside of the hip socket lies approximately a half inch (one centimeter) from the end of the fallopian tube. The ends of the fallopian tube next to the ovary are like the most delicate flower one can imagine, with many petal-like protrusions, called fimbriae, that lay over part of the ovary. The job of the fimbriae is to grasp the one-celled egg as it leaves the ovary and guide it down into the fallopian tube so that conception can occur.

In order for that to happen, the tube must be clear (patent) for sperm to travel up and join with the egg that has been "swallowed" by the fimbriae. In a very real sense, the fallopian tube is the place where human life begins. When adhesions form at the proximal or distal end of the fallopian tube, sperm cannot travel through and neither can the egg. Thus, the internal scarring (adhesions) prevents conception from ever occurring.

If there is some scarring but the tube is slightly open, the mother-to-be can become pregnant but risks having an ectopic pregnancy – a pregnancy that remains inside the tube. Trapped by internal scars, the fertilized egg begins to grow inside the tube. This quickly becomes life-threatening for the mother and life-ending for the embryo.

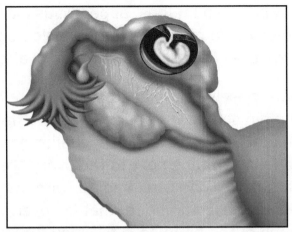

*An ectopic pregnancy occurs when a
fertilized egg becomes stuck in the tube.*

If caught quickly enough, the woman may be given
an injection of methotrexate in order to dissolve the
fertilized egg and end the pregnancy. If the physician
does not diagnose the ectopic pregnancy quickly, the
window for treatment by simple injection will pass. In
that case, the woman must undergo surgery to open the
tube and remove the fertilized egg that has been trapped
in the tube. The surgery often damages the delicate
structures within the fallopian tube. In some cases, the
doctor may recommend removing the tube completely.

In our published studies, tubes that have been treated
surgically have a 35% chance of being opened with
a manual physical therapy, while tubes that have not
undergone surgery have a nearly 70% chance for
success. We believe the lower success rate for tubes that
have been surgically altered is due to the presence of
post-surgical adhesions.

Hydrosalpinx (Swollen Tubes)

When a tube becomes blocked or compromised at the distal end (near the ovary), infection will sometimes occur within the tube itself. Just as your knee can swell when you hurt it, the inside of the tube can swell and fill with liquid. This condition is called a hydrosalpinx.

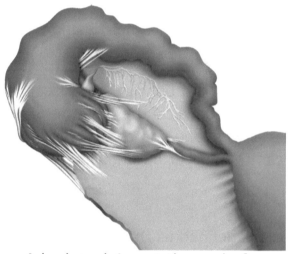

A hydrosalpinx at the end of a
fallopian tube.

Besides the total or near blockage at the end of the tube, a hydrosalpinx can cause three problems.

1.   The tiny fimbriae, whose job is to assist an egg in traveling down toward the uterus, can become glued together by adhesions, rendering them ineffective.

2.   Like a river that has a dam, there is no obvious flow within the swollen tube. Lost in the fluid, the sperm

and egg do not follow their normal direction down to the uterus. This decreases the chance for sperm to meet egg and increases the likelihood of an ectopic pregnancy if they do meet.

3.   Many physicians are concerned that some of the liquid may spill down into the uterus. If it contains an infectious process, that liquid could be harmful to the fertilized egg. Thus, physicians may suggest removing a tube with a hydrosalpinx rather risking the problems described above.

In our experience, if a tube with a hydrosalpinx is opened with a non-surgical physical therapy, the tube generally returns to its prior shape and often its prior function. Pregnancy can then occur naturally, or via IVF.

Endometriosis

Endometriosis is defined as the presence of endometrial tissue, which normally leaves a woman's body during each menstrual period, outside of the uterus. With endometriosis, this tissue can be found in any part of the body, generally in the interstitial spaces – those areas between muscles, organs and connective tissues.

Physicians do not know what causes endometriosis. One theory is that retrograde menstruation flows up through the uterus and tubes, and into a woman's body. This might occur naturally or due to an injury. For example, just before a woman's period, she fell or experienced

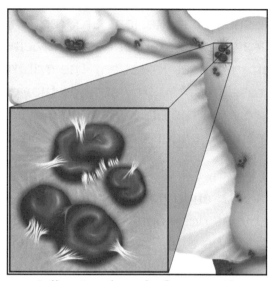

Adhesive bonds frequently attach to endometrial implants.

a trauma to her pelvis that pushed menstrual fluid out of her tubes, past her ovaries and into the interstitial spaces of her body. There is also some indication that endometriosis is hereditary for some women. Environmental factors are also being explored as a cause or contributor to endometriosis in some women.

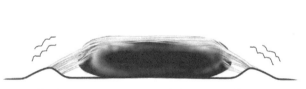

Pain can occur when swelling endometrial tissue pulls on the underlying tissues.

No matter the cause, it is generally accepted that endometrial tissue and adhesions are frequently found together. Wherever endometrial tissue attaches to a structure, it often causes irritation. The irritation causes collagenous crosslinks, the tiny strands that comprise adhesions, to form in the area. As a result, adhesions develop between the endometrial tissue and underlying structure.

Some patients with endometriosis respond well to manual physical therapy, as documented in numerous studies and case reports. We theorize that the following occurs, decreasing pain and improving function in these women.

We know that wherever endometrial tissues land, strands of adhesions often form. As shown in the prior illustrations, these strands can pull on underlying structures when tissues swell during menstruation, causing pain. We have found that a site specific manual therapy appears to detach the crosslinks from the endometrial tissue or the underlying structure. Freed of these strong ropelike bonds, endometrial tissue is free to swell and shrink as menstruation comes and goes, without pulling on the underlying structures and causing pain.

Medical Treatment of Endometrial Pain

Medical treatments vary significantly. Many physicians will begin by prescribing hormone medications such as birth control pills to completely stop the menstrual cycle.

This generally does decrease or stop the pain because the endometrial tissue is no longer swelling. However, this approach is not appropriate if the patient wishes to become pregnant.

Surgery is another option commonly offered by gynecologists. In fact, most physicians will not give a diagnosis of endometriosis without first performing a surgery during which they can visualize endometrial implants. As we saw in previous chapters, the exploratory surgery can cause more adhesions to form, perpetuating the pain or making it worse for some women.

Some surgeons use a Helica or other type of laser to scan only the surface of the endometrial implants. Others tend to burn or cut them away. In some cases, surgeons may be more aggressive, with more extensive cutting that goes deeper within the organs and structures to which the implants are attached. While this may help rid the body of endometriosis, the benefits should be weighed against the damage caused to the organs and the formation of subsequent adhesions. Because adhesions form after most pelvic surgeries, post-surgical adhesion pain becomes a concern for these women.

Endometriosis and Infertility

Endometrial tissue can become glue-like, especially when accompanied by adhesions. Together, adhesions and endometrial tissues can bind structures in the reproductive system, or glue them to other structures.

When they form at the ends of the fallopian tubes, they can block the tubes or cause the delicate fimbria to club together, like a flower with its petals closed. Using even the most sophisticated surgical procedure, it becomes nearly impossible to excise the delicate fingers of the fimbria from the morass of adhesions and endometriosis that forms at the end of the tubes – without causing the scarring (adhesions) from closing the tube again as it heals from the surgery.

Endometriosis can glue the uterus to the bowel (intestine) or the bladder, causing unnatural pulls at the back or front of the uterus. Thus, the uterus can go into spasm or be restricted by these naturally occurring glue-

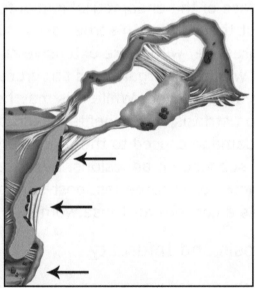

Spasm of the uterus caused by endometriosis and adhesions can cause pain, or decrease fertility.

like bonds – certainly not the most conducive state for implantation. Symptoms and pain can also occur in the bowel or bladder in these cases.

Additional Symptoms of Endometriosis and Accompanying Adhesions

Endometrial implants that form between the uterus and the bladder, which sits in front of the uterus, can also cause a need to urinate frequently. Adhesions that form around a woman's bladder may squeeze it like a straitjacket, decreasing the volume that the bladder can hold and causing an unnatural state of tension.

Polycystic Ovarian Syndrome (PCOS)

PCOS is a condition in which a substance resembling collagen fibers, the building blocks of adhesions, can create a blanket that covers the ovaries. This blanket of collagen often accompanies elevated levels of male hormones. Both of these effects make it difficult for eggs to mature, to leave the ovary, and to proceed to the fallopian tube for fertilization.

The surgical approach to treating PCOS involves either drilling holes in the blanket of collagen or performing a procedure called ovarian wedging. In that surgery, a pie shaped wedge is cut out of the ovary, leaving the inner surfaces exposed. This helps the eggs to exit the ovary and helps decrease the excessive levels of male hormones frequently seen with PCOS.

These surgeries, which may damage or remove a significant portion of the ovary, cause adhesions to form as the body heals from the surgery. Recent studies of a manual physical therapy, examined later in this book, show promising results decreasing adhesions and improving fertility rates for some women with PCOS.

Hormonal Problems

Reproductive physicians recognize an important communication loop in a woman's reproductive cycle, called the pituitary-hypothalamus-ovarian (PHO) axis.

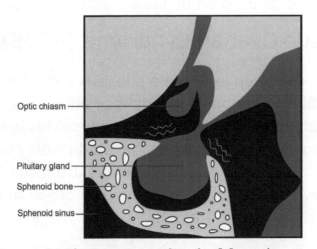

Optic chiasm

Pituitary gland

Sphenoid bone

Sphenoid sinus

As the master gland of female reproduction, the pituitary is housed in a cave like structure, deep in the cranium.

As each menstrual cycle approaches, the ovaries in the pelvis call on the pituitary and hypothalamus glands in the cranium to release follicle-stimulating hormone (FSH) to help eggs mature in preparation for release into the fallopian tube. As a woman ages and approaches menopause, her ovaries require more and more FSH in order to help her eggs mature.

FSH levels are fairly consistent and can be measured on days 2 through 5 of a woman's menstrual cycle. Thus, physicians measure hormonal capacity to conceive with a mature egg and maintain a pregnancy in large part based on day 2 to 5 FSH levels.

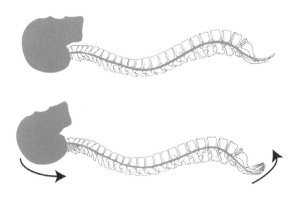

Treatment at the coccyx can sometimes relieve tight areas in the back, neck or head.

Clinical and laboratory values can vary slightly, but when FSH levels are below 10 mIu/ml (milli-international units per milliliter), a woman is generally judged to be hormonally fertile. When FSH levels climb above 10, she is considered by many reproductive physicians to be subfertile or infertile. FSH levels at day 2 to 5 that are at or above 25 mIu/ml are generally considered menopausal. Many reproductive physicians will not treat a woman whose FSH levels are consistently above 10. In some cases, doctors refuse IVF to patients whose FSH levels have ever been at a level of 10 or higher.

Until recently, no natural treatment has been shown to improve FSH levels and fertility in women who were diagnosed subfertile or infertile due to high FSH. Promising results from early studies, examined later in this book, indicate successful outcomes for about half the women who present with high FSH after they have undergone a non-surgical therapy program.

How a Manual Therapy May Help

Like bark surrounds a tree trunk, a strong collagenous structure surrounds the spinal cord. Strong attachments run from the tailbone (coccyx) up the inside of the spine and surround the spinal cord, all the way to the base of the skull. While there are attachments at the base of the skull, the rest of this sheathing,

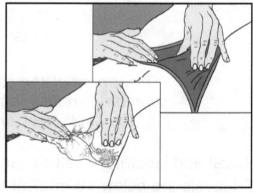

Our manual therapy has been shown to improve fertility.

called the dura, sweeps into the inside of the head

through a hole in the base of the skull called the *foramen magnum*. Once inside the skull, collagenous fibers from this covering (the *dura)* spread throughout the cranium, surrounding and infusing with virtually every cell in the head and brain.

The collagen fibers (fascia) attach to cranial bones and completely surround the pituitary and hypothalamus. Clinically, we have noted that an injury or surgery at the pelvis that pushes or pulls the tailbone forward can create a downward pressure through the dura, to the base of the skull. When this happens, it can pull on the delicate cranial bones that closely encase the pituitary gland. When this physical pressure from the coccyx to the skull is relieved, clinical data indicates that the pituitary and hypothalamus appear to function better, and that FSH levels decrease. For many of the women diagnosed with high FSH, natural fertility followed.

Clinical trials have indicated that relieving pressure at the cranium may improve hormone levels and increase fertility.

Secondary and Unexplained Infertility

C-section is one of the most common major surgeries performed in the Western world. While the surgery may make birth easier for the fetus and less painful for the mother, cutting through the epidermis, the dermis, the pelvic and abdominal muscles, the peritoneum (which encases and protects major abdominal and pelvic organs) and then the uterus requires a significant amount of post-surgical healing.

There is little debate that C-section is a major surgery. Adhesions form as a natural part of the healing process.

Many women are surprised to find that after an initial birth, especially via C-section, sex becomes painful and fertility is decreased or eliminated.

Similarly, a fall onto the back or hip, a pelvic injury or any abdominal or pelvic infection or surgery will create adhesions as the body begins to heal. The delicate tissues of the female reproductive structure cannot function well when they are bound by adhesions. Thus, the woman is diagnosed subfertile or infertile, with secondary or unexplained infertility.

If diagnostic imaging or medical tests are inconclusive or fail to identify the cause of infertility, it is useful to review the patient's history and consider whether adhesions or micro-adhesions may be present, causing the infertility.

Pre-IVF

In vitro fertilization (IVF) is a remarkable process in which eggs are extracted from a woman, combined with her partner's sperm, and then returned into her reproductive tract. We have already seen that the female reproductive tract is subject to adhesions. Adhesions in the reproductive tract can greatly decrease the efficiency, capability and proper function of the female reproductive organs. Recent studies show that therapy to decrease adhesions performed before IVF transfer significantly improved IVF success rates in all age categories. Improvements were profound in women age 38 and above, and roughly three to five times the norm for women 40 or older. Acupuncture has also been beneficial to IVF cycles in some studies.

Adhesions can form at the cervix at the very entrance to the uterus. There they can squeeze the cervix shut or narrow and stiffen the opening like a funnel or an hourglass, making IVF transfer difficult.

Adhesions at the cervix can also create a pull up into the uterus. For example, adhesions that pull the cervix back and to the left can exert unnatural pulls on the uterus each time a woman steps her left foot forward. This can result in uterine spasm or inflammation, which decreases the chance for effective or lasting embryo implantation. Over time, this recurring pull can cause adhesions to form within the uterus. A uterus that is in spasm or is restricted by adhesions is not as effective and does not provide as hospitable an environment for implantation as one that is mobile and unbound, as it is designed to be.

We have seen in the last sections that adhesions can affect hormone levels. A woman's reproductive cycle is a delicate blend of both mechanical and hormonal function. If the mechanics of the glands that regulate hormone production are not in sync, it can be very difficult for fertilization to occur.

Recent studies on increasing IVF success rates, which examine three natural approaches, are promising. One of these approaches addresses adhesions; others do not.

- Psychological group counseling is believed to help relax the body, relieve stress, and make the mind more receptive to fertility, increasing natural pregnancy rates.

- Acupuncture is thought to improve the *chi* or flow of inner energy within the body. In two separate studies, acupuncture has been shown to increase IVF pregnancy rates.

- In several studies a manual physical therapy that directly addresses adhesions has been shown to increase both natural and IVF pregnancy rates by decreasing adhesions in the reproductive tract.

Pain and Women's Health

A common complaint we hear from female patients is that they have been told "Most women hurt" or "You're a woman; it's normal for you to have pain."

While pain may be natural, there is certainly nothing normal about it. Pain is your body's way of telling you that something is wrong. There's always a reason for pain, and in our experience, pelvic pain is not generally found "in the head." It tends to be exactly where the patient feels it, deep within her pelvis.

Some of the reasons women can have pain include these three pertinent facts:

1. A woman's internal environment is open to objects from the outside world. The vagina is a warm, moist, dark environment that is perfect to for bacterial growth. When a woman inserts a tampon or other object (including her partner) in her vagina, she is inserting all of the microbes and bacteria from the outside world that are present on that object. When they come in contact with the rich environment of the vaginal walls, they tend to proliferate.

Even an undetected sub-clinical infection can cause a healing response in the body. As we now know, the first step in healing is the formation of collagen crosslinks the building blocks of adhesions. As these tiny but powerful bonds form on delicate vaginal tissues designed to be supple and mobile, they lose their mobility. As these bonds pull on sensitive structures, they can cause pain.

2. Women who have endometriosis and its frequent companion, adhesions, often go undiagnosed for years. The North American Endometriosis Association found that the average time for a woman with endometriosis to get a diagnosis is more than nine years. Because adhesions do not appear on any non-invasive diagnostic tests, women can have pain from the bonds created by

endometrial tissues or adhesions, conditions that are so often found together, without a definitive diagnostic test. The pain can occur at the first menstruation or later in life. It can persist for years before any surgical procedure is performed to identify the condition or address the endometrial implants and adhesions.

3. Women are the family's main caretaker. Many men will admit, "I have to be nearly dead to go to the doctor."

In general, women appear to be much more diligent about taking of themselves and their family than men. When a woman feels something is amiss in her body, she is often compelled to take action. She may take or apply a medication, or call her physician. In many cases, this leads to a diagnostic surgery to visualize the problem. As we have seen, surgeries create adhesions in the majority of cases – a fact that is well documented in medical literature.

Because endometriosis and adhesions are not visible on most diagnostic tests (X-ray, CT scan or MRI) and can only be visualized during surgery, many women undergo surgeries suggested by their physicians in order to diagnose the problem. As we saw in Chapter Two, adhesions almost always form after pelvic and abdominal surgeries. Thus, the surgery to see what is causing the pain may itself cause additional pain. For many women we have treated, this starts a recurring cycle of pain, surgery and adhesions, with no end in sight. By the time they begin to understand their predicament, they will have been in pain for years or decades. Eventually, they realize that adhesions, which are so often caused by surgeries, are a primary cause of their pain.

Menstrual Pain

Adhesions and endometriosis are not the only cause of menstrual pain. Conditions such as pelvic inflammatory disease, infections, surgeries, falls or abuse elicit healing events, with adhesion formation as their side effect.

Gynecologists regularly monitor the complex hormonal balances and imbalances that occur within a woman's body. However, when no other cause for menstrual pain can be found, it is reasonable for the patient to look back at her history and ask "Have I ever experienced an infection, injury, accident, or repeated blows to that area?"

In looking at her history, she may find healing events that she never considered. One patient told us, "I've never been sick, or had a surgery or trauma. My life has been pretty uneventful as far as anything that would cause adhesions." Upon closer review of her medical history, we learned that she was a gymnast, with recurring falls onto her bottom, hips and pelvis. Years later, she developed pain and infertility due to the internal scars that formed in her youth.

Cheerleaders, especially fliers who are tossed in the air

(and sometimes dropped), track athletes, ice and roller skaters, cyclists and horseback riders often experience injury to their tailbones. As they grow past adolescence into young womanhood, they realize they are having significantly more pain than their peers.

Examine your history for injuries, falls, accidents, infections or surgeries. Unexplained pelvic pain is often caused by adhesive bonds, small but powerful 'straitjackets' that squeeze the delicate and sensitive structures of your reproductive system and/or bowel.

Pain After C-Section or Hysterectomy

While C-sections and hysterectomies are common procedures, they are certainly major surgeries. In both cases, the surgeon is cutting through several layers of tissue to remove either organs or a baby, exposing your well protected, inner-most body to the outside

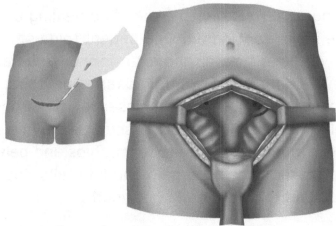

C-section is a major surgery.

environment and then re-closing the body, stitching the remaining tissues back together. Although common, these are major invasive surgeries that require a significant amount of collagen cross-linking to form, from the surface of the skin to the deepest parts of the reproductive system, in order to heal. If the collagen network spreads beyond the cut areas and binds or restricts structures deep within the pelvis, it can cause pain, infertility or digestive problems.

C-Section

In a C-section, the surgeon cuts through the outer layers of the skin, the inner layers, the protective peritoneum, the abdominal muscles and the uterus. The doctor may use an extractor to hold the skin back in order to remove the infant. Then, the surgeon sews the tissues back together, from the inside out.

It is remarkable to consider that C-section is one of the most common major surgeries performed in the western world. If you had one or more C-sections and are experiencing chronic pelvic pain that began within a year or two after the procedure, the cause of your pain may be adhesions that formed naturally to help you heal from the surgery. Post-surgical adhesions can also squeeze the intestines, making the passage of food difficult and causing various abdominal problems – including constipation, diarrhea, or even life-threatening bowel obstructions – in women who have had a C-section.

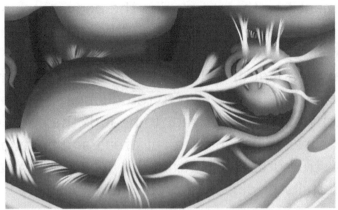

C-section is a common cause of pelvic adhesions and pain.

Hysterectomy

Symptoms after a hysterectomy may be similar to those suffered by women who have pain after a C-section. Whether the hysterectomy is done via open surgery through a horizontal line cut on the front of the pelvis or the uterus is pulled out through the vagina, the trauma of cutting deeply into the body and the inner organs to remove them creates a significant healing event. Adhesive crosslinks rush in to help the body heal after such an event. Once healed, the area can become tight and bound from the adhesions, causing chronic pelvic pain and/or dysfunction that can last a lifetime. If adhesions spread to the front of the nearby vertebrae, pain can occur in the lower back as well.

Pain With Intercourse (Dyspareunia)

Intimacy with her partner should be one of the most

pleasurable events in a woman's life. When she cannot have pleasure with sex or cannot have intercourse at all due to pain at initial penetration, during intercourse or with deep penetration, it can impact her life significantly. These three distinct types of pain can completely stop intimacy with the one she loves; it can make her partner sad, angry, resentful or bitter. It can eliminate the chance for motherhood, end a relationship and even terminate a marriage.

In 2006, we addressed a group of physicians at the American Society for Reproductive Medicine (ASRM) about our scientific findings on reversing intercourse pain and improving sexual function by decreasing adhesions. Approximately 90% of the audience consisted of psychiatrists and psychologists, who were surprised to learn that there is a physical reason for intercourse pain beyond "It's all in the patient's head."

Let's clear this up first – intercourse pain is generally not in your head; it's right where you feel it, at the entrance or deep within your vagina – or both.

Pain at the Entry (Introitus)

The entry to a woman's vagina is subject to pain and healing events due to injury or trauma directly to the area or to nearby areas. Horseback riders, cheerleaders, athletes who sustain blows to their tailbone, and those women who develop vaginal or bladder infections often report pain with initial penetration.

The problem is that the body needs to heal from any of these events. A direct or indirect blow to the tailbone will often cause adhesions to form at the ligaments that attach to the reproductive structures. As crosslinks begin to form within these ligaments, they can pull on the delicate structures of the vagina or reproductive system, causing pain.

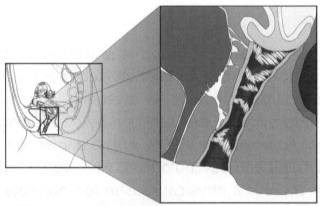

*We often find adhesions have formed
on the vaginal wall.*

An infection in the vagina that spreads to the entry or the labia can cause crosslinks to form in those delicate tissues. Like tiny straitjackets that attach cells to each other within the delicate tissues, these strands of collagen can restrict the normal pliability of the tissues so they cannot expand and move aside during intercourse as they were designed. These constraints exert a pull on the delicate nerves that should be giving pleasure. Thus, the woman experiences significant pain at the precise time she should be having great pleasure.

Pain Within the Vagina

Vaginal, bladder or yeast infections can cause adhesive crosslinks to form on the interior vaginal walls. Sent by the body to help contain and isolate the infection so it does not spread further, these strands lie down on the delicate tissues of the vaginal wall to blanket the area as the first step in the healing process. Once the infection has passed, these strands often remain on the vaginal walls like glue, binding neighboring cells and nerves that should move freely over each other.

During intercourse, the partner's pressure on these delicate nerves can cause significant pain in one or more areas.

When a woman tells her partner about it, he may think she has lost interest in sex or in her partner. When she tells her doctor about it, the doctor may examine her but cannot see the microscopic crosslinks, the building blocks of adhesions, that attach like a thin, invisible sheet of glue to the inner walls of the vagina.

"There's nothing there," the doctor may say. "I think you need to relax. If you like I can refer you to a psychologist or a psychiatrist."

In addition to being inaccurate, this information can be devastating to the patient, who is suffering very real physical pain. She may start questioning whether a psychological issue is causing her condition. "Am I crazy?" she asks herself.

Deep inside however, she knows that this cannot all be "in my head." Meanwhile, her partner believes she does not want to be intimate and her doctor is saying there is nothing there.

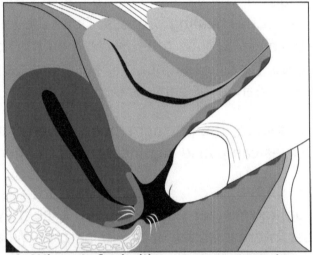

When it feels like your partner is hitting something, he generally is. Usually, we find it is a forward coccyx or an adhered cervix.

Clearly, this situation can cause significant emotional distress in addition to the pain. The time that should bring the greatest pleasure in life causes pain in many women. Like the powerful threads of a nylon rope, microscopic collagen crosslinks, the building blocks of adhesions, are causing the unexplained pain.

It's not that there is no reason for the pain. It is called "unexplained" because the doctors cannot see it! Yet the adhesions remain as a powerful physical presence, preventing pleasure while causing pain, confusion, and heartache.

Pain With Deep Penetration

"It feels like my husband is hitting something," the patient says to her doctor, "during the deepest part of our lovemaking."

Similar to other complaints of pain with intercourse, there are very real physical reasons why this occurs. Pain with deep penetration is not in a woman's head; it occurs in some of the deepest regions of her body accessible to the outside world. There are two main reasons we see pain with deep penetration: anteverted coccyx (forward tailbone) and cervical stenosis (stiffness at the cervix).

Forward Tailbone

From the earliest years of our lives, falls onto our tailbone are common occurrences. For some of us, we may land on the cushy muscles of our bottom and do no damage. But, in other cases, a single traumatic fall landing directly on the tailbone or a series of repeat traumas, such as from horseback or bicycle riding, can cause a state of inflammation at the tailbone.

As we have seen, the body's response to inflammation is

to create tiny but powerful crosslinks. These microscopic strands blanket the area, attaching to any and all structures that are inflamed from the trauma. Adhesions begin to form.

Once our body has healed, the crosslinks remain in the body like glue, attaching to the ligaments that support and maintain the normal, mobile midline position of the tailbone. When this happens, the glue-like bonds can pull the tailbone forward or to one side, preventing it from extending back. Unable to move out of the way, the coccyx is repeatedly struck by the woman's partner during intercourse.

Symptoms of a Forward Tailbone

Constipation can occur, because the passage to eliminate waste is partially blocked during bowel movements.

Pain with deep penetration during sex is common because the tailbone is now curled forward. Being in the way, the partner can no longer glide past it and is repeatedly hitting it.

Difficulty sitting for prolonged periods may occur due to the continuous pressure on this already inflamed area from sitting for an hour or more at a time. This patient will find herself wanting to favor one side or another, rather than sitting directly and symmetrically in her chair. In some cases, the patient finds it uncomfortable to sit at all.

Pain in the lower back or at the base of the skull is an unexpected but very real side-effect of a malaligned or forward positioned tailbone. The coccyx is the very bottom attachment of the strong structure called the dura, which surrounds the spinal cord. The dura ascends from the tailbone to the sacrum, then all the way up to the base of the skull. In some patients, a forward tailbone will pull down on the dura, causing pain in the lower back and/or at the base of the skull, due to the physical pull.

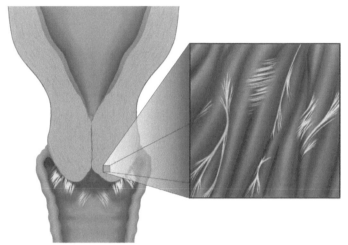

Adhesions at the cervix (front view).

We find a forward tailbone is often the missing link in severe or recurring headaches. If the tailbone is pulling the dura down, the base of the skull can also be pulled down by this pressure. Thus, many patients will continue to have headaches unless the tailbone is brought back into proper alignment by freeing the ligaments of the adhesions that are shortening them, and returning the coccyx to its normal, mobile position.

Cervical Stenosis (Stiff Cervix)

Vaginal infections, even undiagnosed subclinical infections, cause healing events to occur. The first step in healing is for the body to send in crosslinks, the building blocks of adhesions, to surround and isolate the infected area. This process of isolation makes it easier for our white blood cells and immune system to continue the healing process.

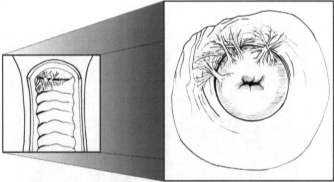

Vaginal or bladder infections can cause adhesions that migrate to the cervix, causing pain with deep intercourse.

Once healing has occurred, these crosslinks tend to remain in place, often binding the cells within the cervix together. This can happen deep within the cervix, not only on the surface. Bound in this way, the cells of the cervix are pulled forward, backwards, to the side or simply squeezed together, creating mal-alignment and stiffness (stenosis).

Three Main Consequences of a Stenosed Cervix

1. Pain. Having lost their usual mobility, the bound cells within the cervix move as a unit. When they are forced to move during intercourse, a pull is exerted onto the nerves in the cervix, which can cause pain.

2. Difficulty for sperm to access the uterus. Some patients with stenosed cervices report that their reproductive physician has difficulty inserting a catheter past the cervix and into the uterus during *in vitro* fertilization (IVF) or intrauterine insemination (IUI). Naturally, this same difficulty can hinder a woman's ability to conceive naturally, as sperm have difficulty entering a tight or partially closed cervix.

3. Adhesions in the uterus. When the cervix is adhered, it can cause problems further up in the uterus. For example, if a cervix is adhered and pulled back and to the left, every step forward that woman takes with her left leg can pull on the cervix, causing a repetitive pull up into the uterus. Some women do not notice this; others report feeling a pulling sensation or pain on one side. With these repeated pulls caused by normal walking, the uterus becomes inflamed on that left side and adhesions form in response to the inflammation. The result is that adhesions can form within the uterus or on the uterine wall, causing spasm and sometimes pain, and deterring fertility.

In some cases, we have seen blocked fallopian tubes on

the side where the cervix has been pulled forward. Unless these adhesions at the cervix are freed, this condition will persist, creating an inhospitable surface for implantation – as well as causing infertility due to tubal occlusion (blockage).

Decreased Sexual Response

We had only been treating pelvic pain and blocked fallopian tubes for a few women when patients began calling with unusual responses.

"It's a bit embarrassing to talk about," the woman said, "but ever since you treated me, I have been having orgasms like I never had in my life before. It's been just such a remarkable response – I wanted to call and let you know."

After a dozen women reported such results, we discussed it with our medical director, a research gynecologist.

"That's really important" he said. "We need to conduct a study on this."

With his encouragement, we conducted and published the first of several studies on increasing desire, arousal, lubrication and orgasm in women using a manual physical therapy. We presented this data to a large medical conference (the American Society for Reproductive Medicine) in 2006. The study was considered significant because no other medical treatment has been scientifically shown to increase every measurable domain of sexual function.

When we began our sexual function research, we approached this area with a significant amount of caution given the sensitive nature of the subject and the many unsubstantiated claims of products to improve sex. Several of our patients were reporting much better sex and the gynecologist, who was Chief of Staff at a local hospital, insisted that our findings were important. Thus, we began investigating why patients we were treating for adhesions were reporting significant improvements in sexual response.

We used the Female Sexual Function Index (FSFI) to measure our results. This is a validated scientific test of the six major domains of sexual function: desire, arousal, lubrication, orgasm, satisfaction and pain.

As we now know, when a woman has a vaginal infection, even a subclinical one, tiny strands of collagen called crosslinks develop on the surface of the vagina to help stop the spread of that infection to other areas. When this occurs, the microscopic adhesions – so small that they are often invisible to gynecologists – can blanket the delicate nerves that cause pleasure and excite the lubricating glands of the reproductive tract. When this happens, any of the responsive functions noted above can be affected, with or without accompanying pain.

Your partner may wonder what is going on due to your

loss of interest in sex. Your gynecologist examines you and does not find a problem. Yet, with all the hype and circumstance you see in the media about sex, you just don't feel it, or worse, you feel pain.

Structurally, the clitoris is a major structure for sexual arousal. Analogously, if the clitoris were a tree, the G-spot would be the root of the tree. This is generally about 1.5 inches (4 centimeters) inside the vagina within the anterior (front) vaginal wall. Clinically, we find this to be an area where tiny adhesive bonds frequently form due to infection. When that occurs, a blanket of collagen fibers, invisible to the human eye, can dull sexual response by covering the nerve endings that should be firing with pleasure during intercourse.

No medical, surgical or pharmaceutical intervention has been shown to adequately address this structural problem. In order to reverse the situation and increase those responses, we find that these tiny mechanical bonds need to be freed mechanically, with a non-surgical therapy.

CHAPTER 7
PUBLISHED DATA

Research on Nonsurgical Treatments

History of our Research

Our research efforts began in the early 1990s, when we started seeing some remarkable results decreasing adhesions in patients with chronic pain. We were treating a workers' compensation patient for a pelvic injury when she told us she was shocked, because she became pregnant.

The patient reported having blocked fallopian tubes for seven years, used no birth control and had the same boyfriend this entire time. The only thing that was different was that we treated her with the therapy we developed to decrease adhesions.

Hearing about that, a physician referred four other women during the next year. Two came with totally blocked fallopian tubes; it was medically impossible for them to conceive naturally. The other two had been infertile for several years, and had given up on medical treatments. Three of the women became pregnant, including the two with totally blocked tubes.

Then the physician referred his wife, who had been infertile for 11 years. She also had significant pain from endometriosis. "If you can just help her pain, that would be great," the doctor said. His wife was 41 years old at the time.

In truth, we were not trying to open her fallopian tube. She only had one tube and that had been blocked for 11 years. Her gynecologic file was an inch and a half thick, due to all the surgeries she had endured. One day, she came in and said "Belinda, I'm not sure whether to hug you or punch you; before you treated me, I was totally infertile. Now I'm going to be 42 – and I'm pregnant!"

Taken together, we felt these were important cases. We knew we needed to share them but we knew nothing about research. About that time, Gerald Wiechmann, PhD, a senior researcher at the National Institutes of Health, heard about our success from his son, a radiologist in our hometown of Gainesville, Florida. The son had apparently viewed several of the pre- and post-therapy dye tests, and mentioned the results to his father – who became fascinated. Together with Dr. Wiechmann, we published a small in-house study in 1997 revealing infertility reversals in a number of women, some with blocked tubes, some without. At this point we began to understand the scientific method.

In the scientific method, you can start when you have seen unusual results in a single patient; then you attempt the same treatment on other patients with similar conditions, and keep track of the results. If you see positive results in a number of patients, you try to develop an objective test to measure and validate your results. Thankfully, such a test already existed for whether or not we could open blocked fallopian tubes, so we could see successes and failures clearing them, using before and after dye tests.

When we shared our results among the gynecologists in our medically oriented town of Gainesville, Florida (home of the University of Florida Medical School) the chief of staff of the hospital called us in.

"What's this about opening blocked fallopian tubes?" he asked. Larry handed Dr. King half a dozen charts of women whose tubes we had opened. He opened one chart, then another . . . then another. "Good grief" he said "you are doing things with your hands I'm not sure I could do surgically – and I am very good surgeon. This is extraordinary."

He turned to look me in the eye and asked "Are you doing any research on this work?"

"No," I answered.

"Would you like to?" he asked.

"Yes, I suppose we would, but we know very little about research," I said.

"I'll tell you what," he said. "If you'd like to do some research I will be your research director. I won't charge you a dime; I believe this is important work. The world needs to know about this." Thus our efforts in research began.

Blocked fallopian tubes ended up being a perfect condition to research because we had films taken by an independent radiologist before we treated women showing total blockage. Then we could treat, and have films taken by another radiologist afterwards (unless the woman became pregnant beforehand.) If the "after" films showed that a tube opened or the woman became pregnant, we knew were successful in opening her tubes. If the "after" films showed persistent blockage, we knew that we weren't successful. Thus, we could begin to tabulate results in a scientific manner.

In this vein, we began to publish research in treating blocked fallopian tubes, female infertility, sexual problems, endometriosis pain and small bowel obstructions over the next 25 to 30 years. In female infertility, this culminated in a 2015 study of 1,392 infertile women we had treated. The results of that study are shown below, along with results of some of the other studies published on our work to date.

Overview of our Research

The purpose of this short book was to give a general overview of adhesions: how they form, their structure and anatomy, the difficulty in diagnosing them, and some of the problems they can cause. We gathered this information over the course of 30 years of treating patients with adhesions. We have worked with scientists, physicians, gifted therapists and patients to investigate the too-often-overlooked phenomenon of adhesions in the body.

This chapter presents the results of using the therapy we developed, the Clear Passage Approach (CPA) on a variety of conditions caused, or exacerbated by adhesions. We started collecting data in the mid-1990s after we had noticed positive results that we felt needed to be shared. We began publishing results of our work with an in-house publication on decreasing adhesions and improving fertility, in 1997.

Coached by physicians and scientists at the nearby University of Florida medical school, we followed what is called "the scientific method," which is designed to investigate new phenomena. Using this framework, researchers progress from reporting individual case studies to multiple case studies. If we continued to see good results, we moved on to studies which examine larger populations for safety and efficacy. If those studies show the new method is safe and effective with a particular population or condition, the next step is to conduct controlled studies, comparing treated subjects to non-treated groups, or those who are given sham (fake) treatments.

Because our patients were paying for therapy and had

limited time to succeed, it was deemed unethical to give them sham treatment, so we compared our results to "no therapy" groups. In some cases, we compared them to published studies of accepted medical treatments, such as "standard of practice" infertility treatments such as surgeries, which already had published results.

Thus, our research expanded from our first in-house study in 1997 through a number of case and pilot studies, to our most recent studies on larger patient populations. Over time, we have found that the results from our pilot studies are valid predictors of results we achieve in larger studies.

In the sections below, we present the most recent studies published on a variety of conditions. We did very well with certain conditions, and not with others. Below, we will present all of the results we have at hand, at the time of publication. In all cases, the published data and studies shown below were analyzed and accepted by independent "peer reviewers," physicians and scientists who examine studies for validity, bias, impartiality, and potential to improve medical knowledge, before being accepted for publication.

Where possible, we will give 'whole number' percentage rates for success or failure, followed by the fraction of successes (the numerator, shown as the number above) over the total examined (denominator, below.) For example, 50% (10/20) means we treated 20 patients in this group and 10 had success: thus 50% success rate.

P-value, Odds Ratios (OR), and Confidence Intervals (CI) are shown in some cases for readers who understand statistical modeling. In general, the lower the P-value, the greater the validity; anything smaller than P=0.05 is usually considered scientifically valid. OR and CI require explanation beyond this author's ability to simplify; the scientists affiliated with our studies advised us that our OR and CI numbers are very good.

Infertility: While we began as a clinic treating chronic, debilitating pain, we were surprised when women for whom we were treating pelvic pain reported that we were opening their blocked fallopian tubes. While the only known treatment for this was surgery, it was easy to test whether we were truly helping these women – who were totally infertile due to blocked tubes. It was easy to calculate our results for this; either tubes cleared or they did not, evidenced by a simple dye test (or pregnancy before the test.)

When it became obvious that we were indeed helping open tubes non-surgically, we were encouraged by physicians and patients to branch out into other areas of infertility, and to document areas where we could help. Soon, we began to treat other women with infertility from different causes, such as endometriosis, PCOS, high FSH, etc. When women asked if we could help increase their chances with in vitro fertilization (IVF), we started keeping data on that aspect as well. The more we treated this population, the more we realized that we could offer an effective conservative therapy to women who did not want to undergo a surgery.

Our earliest published studies with infertile women included only small groups of patients. Women in our early studies (natural and pre-IVF) were infertile for an average of 4.5 years (range 1 to 20 years) prior to therapy.

As we progressed over the years, we have reviewed thousands of patient successes and failures in our studies. In a landmark 10-year infertility study published in 2015, we were pleased to find that the results from nearly 1,400 infertile women closely paralleled the results of our earlier pilot studies. Below, we give an overview of our published studies in this area, in an easy to read format.

Bowel obstructions: When people began to read of our success clearing blocked fallopian tubes, several people who suffered recurring small bowel obstructions began contacting us, asking if we could clear their "larger tubes." We had been wondering this ourselves, but it was a bit daunting to move from 'life giving' work returning fertility to infertile women, to 'live saving' work – helping people with life-threatening intestinal obstructions.

In looking at the condition, we learned that intestines (bowels) can become partially or totally blocked with adhesions, creating a terrible quality of life for patients. They were often in pain, had great difficulties with food intake, and were often afraid to go to a friend's house or restaurant for dinner, fearful that an obstruction would occur that would send them to the hospital for surgery – or worse, that they would die. They were afraid to travel, to be too far from their hospital. We would commonly hear "when I look in the mirror every morning, I ask myself 'Is this the day I am going to die?' "

Adding to their problem, the main treatment for bowel obstruction was surgery – which is also the primary cause of bowel obstruction. Thus, many found themselves in an ever-revolving circle of adhesions-obstruction-surgery-adhesions, with no end in sight. Naturally, our hearts went out to these people; we wanted to know if we could help them.

Once again, our research in this area started with small single or multiple case pilot studies. As it became obvious that we could help many of these patients, we began publishing larger studies.

As we go to press, we are submitting a relatively large prospective controlled study of over 200 patients examining the therapy's effectiveness treating people who suffer recurring small bowel obstructions. The results of this study, which compares patients who did and did not receive therapy for recurring bowel obstructions, are remarkably promising. We hope to share those results in the next edition of this book, once that study has been published.

Menstrual and intercourse pain, sexual dysfunction: We began in 1989 as a small clinic designed to treat unexplained chronic pain. That population of patients remains core to the work we love, and still comprises much of our patient base. While tests exist to test 'before and after' results for improving sexual function, the variety of pain problems we treat does not easily allow us to test changes in pain. Thus, while we often see significant turn-arounds, publishing with such a diverse population is problematic, at best. The published data on improvements in sexual function is clear, compelling, and presented below. If you are troubled with chronic pain, we suggest you call for data relative to your needs.

Adhesions, the common factor: In all of these studies, the common factor being studied is the decrease of adhesions via non-surgical manual therapy. Whether we are treating the tiny crosslinks that join individual cells within the uterus or cervix, larger adhesions that squeeze nerves causing pain, or that block organs like the fallopian tubes or intestines, the large rope-like adhesions that bind larger bodily structures together, sometimes pulling the torso forward in people with massive abdominal adhesions – the basic structure of adhesions remains the same. Naturally occurring adhesion formation due to the joining of collagenous crosslinks can create straightjackets within the body, squeezing structures or joining together nearby structures, causing pain and/or dysfunction.

The release of these crosslinks from each other using a natural manual therapy is analogous to pulling apart the run in a three-dimensional sweater, as the adhesions unravel and the body returns to an earlier state of pain-free mobility and function. This deformation of the adhesions is the common factor in all of the studies and conditions in which CPA has improved life for patients.

Where to get therapy: Literally millions of people in the world suffer needlessly with adhesions. There appears to be no end to this problem that plagues patients and their doctors throughout the world. Brilliant and gifted physicians are stymied by adhesion formation after performing their best surgical repairs. In fact, healthcare providers and their families represent our largest population base – fully a third of our patients are doctors, physical therapists, nurses, or their parents, children and spouses, sent to us by their family provider.

There are many gifted manual therapists in the world. Many focus on treating aches and pains in the muscles and joints of our body, while some look at the organs and the problems that may occur due to adhesive restrictions. We do not hold a monopoly on knowledge of treating adhesions, or of helping the viscera – the organs of the body. We are glad to share our knowledge of adhesions and possible cures, as the gift that we leave behind in the world. Our story is unique, due to the decades of experience decreasing adhesions anywhere in the body and treating the conditions listed in this book, non-surgically.

We encourage anyone who believes they may have adhesion-related problems to:

1. Know that the problem is not "all in your head;"

2. Seek help from a healthcare professionals who is familiar with biomechanics of the body and adhesions;

3. If your provider does not understand that adhesions can cause pain and dysfunction as they grow from area to area within the body, find one who does.

4. Make sure that your physician and therapist screen you, to keep you safe with the work your therapist will perform;

5. Get a referral and clearance from your physician before starting any manual therapy regimen.

In the following section, you can examine published results that examine the CPA, for many of the conditions covered in this book. Extrapolated from peer-reviewed journals, these results are divided into three sections, based in part on when we developed the work, and in part on importance to us:

• Female infertility (Giving life)

• Adhesions and small bowel obstructions (Saving lives)

• Pelvic pain and sexual dysfunction (Saving relationships and marriages)

Female Infertility: Giving Life

Study:

Ten-year Retrospective Study on the Efficacy of a Manual Physical Therapy to Treat Female Infertility *Alternative Therapies in Health and Medicine* – 2015

Description:

This landmark study examined the results treating 1,392 infertile women treated with the Clear Passage Approach (CPA) at all of our clinics, between 2002 and 2011.
The study compares success rates of CPA to traditional medical treatments (surgeries and pharmaceuticals).

Results:

Success rates with CPA therapy rivaled or exceeded medical success rates in some common causes of female infertility: Blocked fallopian tubes, endometriosis, PCOS (often accompanied with failure to ovulate), and advanced age, measured by high FSH hormone levels.
In some areas (such as endometriosis) the results were comparable to surgery. In some cases (such as Primary Ovarian failure) we did not do well at all.

Some side-effects of therapy were transient, such as temporary soreness after therapy. Lasting side-effects such as increased desire, lubrication and orgasm, and decreased or eliminated intercourse or menstrual pain are presented separately, in the Sexual Function part of this chapter. Endometriosis pain is presented in both the Infertility and Sexual Function sections.

While the great majority of our successes were natural, the therapy also increased in vitro fertilization (IVF) pregnancy rates significantly in all age groups, when performed before embryo transfer, with fairly dramatic success in women who were nearing the end of their reproductive age. For example, rates in women over 40 were roughly three to five times the norm.

Opening Blocked Fallopian Tubes

Results:

The therapy opened totally blocked fallopian tubes in:

69% of women with no prior tubal surgery (124/180)

35% of women with prior surgery to their tubes (19/55)

61% of women overall (143/235)

60% rate opening blocked fallopian tubes in women with endometriosis (40/67)

In largest published study of its type, CPA therapy

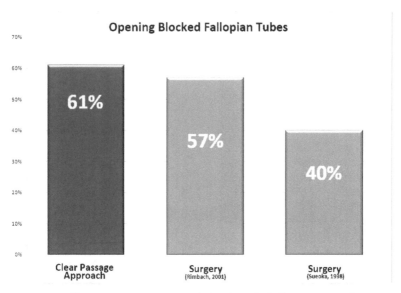

Overall rates opening blocked fallopian tubes

opened totally blocked fallopian tubes in 61% of (143/235) women diagnosed with total tubal occlusion (both tubes blocked) before therapy. Of interest, this rate matched the percentage cited in *Contemporary Ob-Gyn* in 2008, which showed a 61% success rate for CPA opening tubes in (17/28) women in a pilot study conducted seven years earlier.

Success rates in the larger study were 69% for (124/180) for women who had not undergone prior tubal surgery and 35% for (19/55) women who had undergone a prior tubal surgery. The lower rate was surmised to be caused by post-surgical scarring on the delicate fallopian tubes.

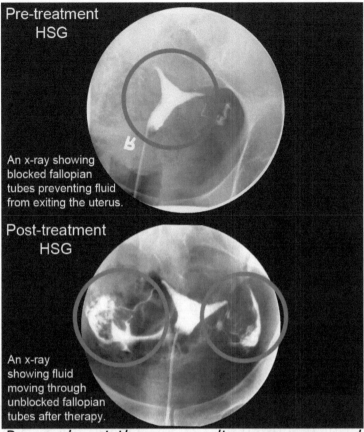

Pre-treatment
HSG

An x-ray showing
blocked fallopian
tubes preventing fluid
from exiting the uterus.

Post-treatment
HSG

An x-ray
showing fluid
moving through
unblocked fallopian
tubes after therapy.

Pre- and post-therapy results were measured by dye tests, surgery or natural pregnancy, which can only occur to open tubes.

Clearing Hydrosalpinx

Results: 45% cleared of hydrosalpinx (47/105)

Per the 10-year study (2015), the CPA opened tubes in 45% (47/105) of women with hydrosalpinx (liquid-filled tubes), a very challenging group. Reproductive physicians often remove tubes with hydrosalpinx, feeling they will never function, yet the therapy returned fertility for many of these women. Interestingly, this rate confirmed the rate of their very first pilot study treating women with hydrosalpinx, presented to the American Society for Reproductive Medicine (ASRM), and published as an abstract in 2006, when the therapy cleared tubes in 50% of women with hydrosalpinx.

Pregnancy Rates for Women With Clear Tubes

Results: 57% (81/143) pregnancy rates after therapy

• 80 natural pregnancies; 1 via IVF

• Several women experienced additional (second or third) natural pregnancies after treatment suggesting the results of therapy can last for many years.

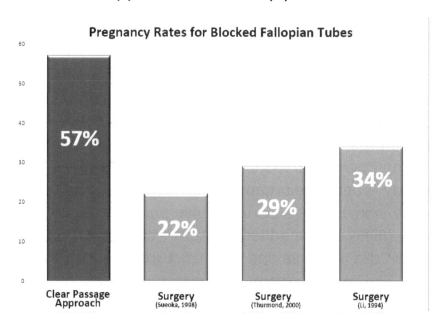

Pregnancy Rates for Blocked Fallopian Tubes

In the large 10-year study, pregnancy rates for women whose tubes were opened by the therapy were 57% (81/143) after therapy (vs. 22% – 34% after surgery)

Notes:

1) Location of the blockage did not influence clearance rates;

2) While surgery can often open tubes that are proximally blocked (near the uterus), surgically opened fallopian tubes tend to close within six months after surgery because of post-surgical scarring. In the largest study ever conducted on follow-up after tubal surgery, a repeat HSG dye test six months after opening tubes by surgery showed a total re-occlusion rate of 81% (35/43), six months after surgery.

Endometriosis - Overview

Endometriosis is a complex condition that contains both mechanical and hormonal elements. In this condition, endometrial tissue that is normally found in the lining of the uterus, and that should be expelled with every menstrual period, is found in the interstitial spaces of the body – between organs, muscles, nerves and bones. When a woman has a period, these endometrial implants swell, pulling on the adhesions that frequently form between the implants and the structure on which they reside. The main concerns for women with endometriosis are

- infertility

- moderate to severe period pain

- moderate to severe pain with intercourse

- decreases sexual function (e.g., desire, lubrication, orgasm)

CPA therapy has been studied in all of these areas. In all cases, the therapy is designed to decrease the cross-linking, the tiny but powerful white attachments shown in the drawing in the chapter covering endometriosis. Below is data on infertility reversal for women we treated with endometriosis. Results of the reversing pain and sexual dysfunction are given later in this chapter.

Endometriosis Related Infertility

Results: 43% (128/299) pregnancy rate

In the 10-year study, the therapy yielded pregnancy rates of 43%, which is comparable to the 38% to 42% success rates of surgeries cited in the study. Therapy avoids the risk and cost of surgery, including anesthesia, inadvertent enterotomy (cutting through or into nearby structures mistakenly), and post-surgical adhesions.

Of the 56 patients with follow-up who underwent IVF post-CPA treatment, the clinical pregnancy rate after transfer was 55.4% (31/56), which is 1.3 times that of the national average of 40.3% for IVF transfer alone in women with endometriosis.

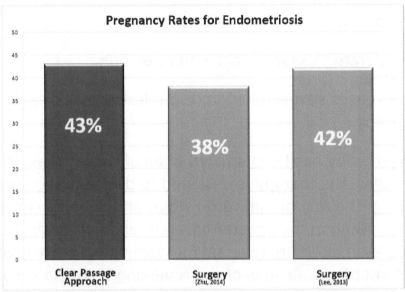

*Pregnancy rates after therapy closely matched
surgical success rates cited in the study*

PCOS - Infertility

Results: 54% (15/28) pregnancy rate

14 natural pregnancies; 1 pregnancy by IVF

In a subset of women experiencing infertility due to
polycystic ovarian syndrome (PCOS), the non-surgical
physical therapy yielded a 54% (15/28) success rate.
While this subset is not large, it is promising. The results
compare well with the 22% to 33% success rates
for medications and surgery, which generally consists
of ovarian drilling (cutting holes through the tissues
surrounding the ovary, and then into the ovary itself) and

ovarian wedging (cutting a wedge-shaped piece out of the ovary.)

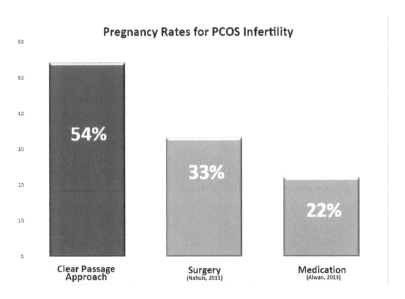

Pregnancy Rates for PCOS Infertility

Clear Passage Approach — 54%
Surgery (Nahuis, 2011) — 33%
Medication (Alwan, 2013) — 22%

<u>Comparison to medications and surgery:</u> According to the study published in 2015: Options for standard medical treatment of PCOS include medications—clomiphene citrate, metformin, or combinations thereof —and surgical interventions to induce ovulation. The rates of pregnancy in patients treated using the CPA were directly compared with success rates for various interventions reported in the literature. The CPA demonstrated significantly higher rates of pregnancy when compared with metformin alone. CPA treatment presented no significant differences in rates of pregnancy when compared with clomiphene citrate or the surgical interventions of ovarian wedging or drilling.

127

High FSH - Hormone Related Infertility

Results:

38% pregnancy rate in our initial pilot, 2009 study (6/16)
All pregnancies were natural in the pilot study

39% pregnancy rate in our large, 2015 study (48/122)
43 pregnancies by natural conception; 5 pregnancies via
IVF

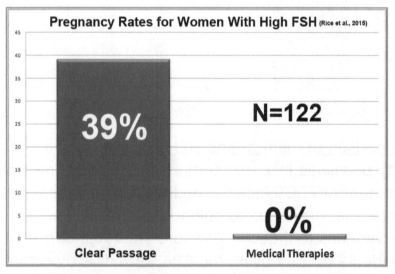

*Pregnancy rates after therapy for women
diagnosed infertile or subfertile due to high FSH.*

CPA therapy improved hormonal fertility for women
with high FSH (follicle stimulating hormone) levels. FSH
levels (measured on Day 2 through 5 of a woman's cycle,
typically rise as a woman approaches menopause. When
FSH levels are above 10 mIU/mL, most reproductive

physicians consider the patient subfertile or infertile. In fact, many reproductive endocrinologists will not consider performing IVF (in vitro fertilization) on a woman with FSH levels at 10 or above. Because no standard medical treatment has been shown to improve fertility in women with high FSH, no comparison could be made between the therapy and standard medical treatments.

In the 10-year study, CPA therapy treated 122 women who were diagnosed subfertile or infertile, due to FSH levels above 10. The therapy, improved FSH levels or yielded pregnancy in 49% of the women, and 39% (48/122) of them became pregnant following therapy; 43 or the pregnancies were natural, and five were by IVF.

Pre-IVF Therapy

Results:

56% pregnancy rate (82/146) for women who had CPA therapy before embryo transfer. This is 1.5 times higher than that of the national average of 37%. (SART 2010 data)

By age, compared to National Success Rates (SART – the Society for Assisted Reproductive Technology.)

Age	With CPA %	Without CPA %	P Value*
Under age 35	68%	45%	.0067
35 through 37	60%	37%	.0133
38 through 40	49%	29%	.0107
41 through 42	54%	29%	.0039
Older than 42	44%	9%	<.0001

Percent of pregnancies using CPA before embryo transfer vs. without CPA

* P-value is a statistical term used to measure results. The P-values above are considered excellent, providing validity to the results.

In these cases, the therapy focused on decreasing adhesions and collagen crosslinking in four areas:

• The uterus and cervix;

• The ovaries and fallopian tubes;

• The dura, the collagenous covering of the spinal cord which runs from the coccyx (tailbone) in the pelvis to the cranial base (at the occiput), then into the cranium;

• At the pituitary and hypothalamus, via the dura and the osseous structures (bones) that comprise the cranium, and encase the pituitary gland.

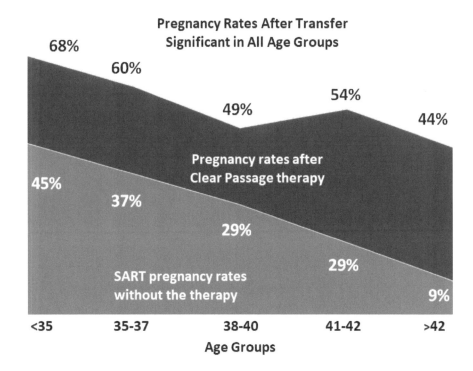

**Pregnancy Rates After Transfer
Significant in All Age Groups**

68%

60%

54%

49%

44%

**Pregnancy rates after
Clear Passage therapy**

45%

37%

29%

29%

**SART pregnancy rates
without the therapy**

9%

| <35 | 35-37 | 38-40 | 41-42 | >42 |

Age Groups

Primary Ovarian Failure - POF

Results:

20% (1/5 patients) pregnancy rate in patients with POF via natural conception

While it is difficult to gather meaningful data from a subset of only five patients, initial results indicate that we do not offer any meaningful improvement for women diagnosed with Primary Ovarian Failure (POF).

Adhesions and Small Bowel Obstructions

Results:

Return to surgery rate within two years: 3% to 7%
Expected rate without Clear Passage: 30%

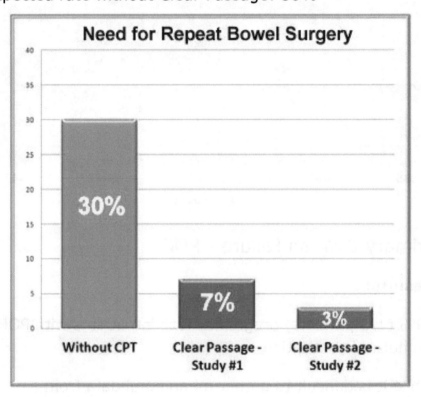

Introduction

With our strong commitment to measuring and publishing results scientifically, bowel obstructions presented several research challenges to us. For one thing, there are 21 feet (7 meters) of small intestine (bowel), *vs.* about four inches (10 cm) of fallopian tubes. Even more challenging, when a tube is blocked, the woman can still function in all other ways. When the bowel is blocked, the patient is in an immediate life-threatening position. The obstruction must clear, or the patient will die. Finally, there are many more co-morbidities in the abdomen and bowel – concurrent conditions we must consider before we put our hands on a person who suffers repeat bowel obstructions.

A major problem for these patients is that the surgery designed to cure or save them often creates new adhesions – that block the bowels months or years later. Repeat surgeries cause repeat obstructions, we (and surgeons) see this every day. No matter how caring and skilled your doctor, surgeons cannot prevent the adhesions that form naturally in the body as it heals from the surgery. Thus, repeat life-threatening obstructions become a way of life for many people. These are the people we tend to help the most.

As usual, we started with publishing interesting case studies, then built into larger groups. As we go to press, we are submitting a controlled study with over 200 subjects in it, half of whom received CPA after bowel obstructions (the Treatment Group), and half of whom did not (the Control Group.) Look for that study to be published in 2018.

The data in this chapter represents the latest clinical data we have as of the date of this writing. It includes "before and after" reports from independent physicians and tests that have been published and validated by independent scientists and physicians.

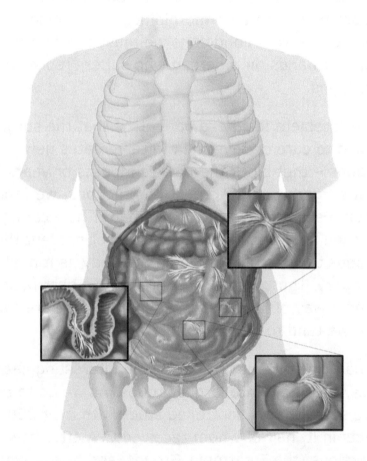

Adhesions may form as curtains or ropes within or between the bowel, completely blocking the passage designed to transport food.

Success Rates Overview

Published studies and statistical data show strong evidence of the improvements that our non-surgical therapy achieves in people with recurring small bowel obstructions (SBO). These include cleared obstructions, cleared strictures, decreased need for medications, decreased pain and improved quality of life. More importantly, they show a dramatic decrease in the need for additional surgery versus the expected rate. Following is a timeline summary of our investigation with these conditions.

2008 – First SBO Patients Treated

When published studies showed we could open fallopian tubes blocked by adhesions, we developed therapy to clear the adhesions that cause bowel obstructions. Our success with these patients came quickly, inspiring us to begin to track data suitable for publication.

2013 – SBO Published Studies

We began publishing case studies about clearing bowel obstructions and adhesions via manual therapy using objective reports from independent physicians noting:

• Before and after x-rays showing cleared bowel obstruction;

• Before and after x-rays showing eliminated stricture (narrowing) in the bowel;

• A patient whose only nutrition was intravenous before therapy could eat normally following therapy.

Clearing Obstructions

Before treatment *After treatment*

Obstruction

No Obstruction

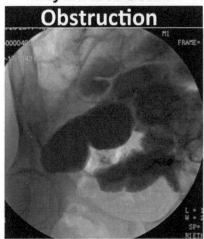 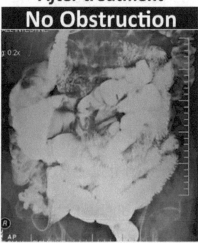

Clearing Bowel Strictures

Before treatment *After treatment*

Stricture

No Stricture

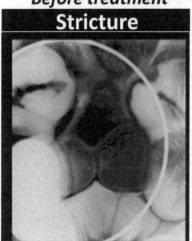 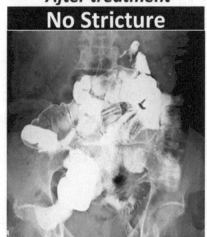

Journal of Clinical Medicine, 2013

2014 –Validated Measurement Test Published

Some patients who have recurring SBOs have other symptoms; others do not. We published a scientifically validated questionnaire to measure common but serious quality of life issues for patients experiencing small bowel obstructions 'before and after' therapy. This test, now available to all physicians and scientists, helped give an overview of 'quality of life' changes for people who suffer repeat obstructions.

2015 – Measuring and Publishing Data on Quality of Life After Therapy

The independent data noted above generated interest in further studies. Subjective data, such as pain relief, is considered relevant when screened using a scientifically validated test, such as the one we published in 2014. We use it to measure:

• Pain presence

• Pain severity

• Gastrointestinal symptoms

• Diet

• Medication

• Quality of life

• Range of motion (prior surgical adhesions can bind the abdomen, restricting trunk mobility)

As a result, we can now identify the areas where we are most effective, shown below.

2015 – Present Data to 15,000 Physicians

We were invited to present our work to 15,000 international gastroenterologists at Digestive Disease Week in Washington D.C. Results of that pilot study were published in the journal *Gastroenterology* (May 2015). Scientists noted improvement in every domain of 'quality of life' measurable for patients with prior bowel obstructions, including:

• Pain decreased in 85% of patients;

• Gastrointestinal symptoms deceased in 73% of patients;

• Diet improved for 100% of patients who reported a severe impact on their diet before therapy, and in 50% of patients overall;

• 83% of patients who were taking medication for bowel function maintenance before therapy were able to completely stop their medication;

• Significant improvements in all six areas of trunk range of motion (flexion, extension, right and left side bending, right and left rotation)

Measuring Repeat Surgeries with and without Therapy

A vital concern for anyone who has ever undergone the terrible ordeal of bowel obstruction surgery is to avoid repeat hospitalization and surgery. Adding to this concern is the fact that abdominal surgery is the primary cause of bowel obstruction. Thus, post-surgical SBO patients worry they will have to undergo one or more repeat surgeries, leaving them in a repeating cycle of obstruction-surgery-adhesions with no end in sight.

We have treated over 400 patients over the last eight years with concerns they would have to undergo another obstruction surgery. This large number allows us to start gathering long-term data on success rates, including percent of return surgeries in our patients compared to those who don't receive our therapy.

We compiled the first of our long-term "return to surgery" rates from two sets of patients who received our therapy, and compared them to the norm (no therapy):

• Dataset #1 – Clinical data on our earliest bowel obstruction patients

• Dataset #2 – Scientific data published in a 2015 medical textbook

Repeat Surgeries without CPA Therapy

Repeat surgery within 30 days: According to U.S.

government statistics, 18% of patients who undergo bowel obstruction surgery are readmitted to the hospital within 30 days after their surgery. Some of these repeat surgeries are due to infection from bowel contents that leaked into the abdominal cavity during the first surgery. Set free in a warm, dark, moist environment, the escaped bacteria can grow quickly, creating an internal infection that requires immediate repeat surgery, with antibiotics administered directly to the surgical site.

Repeat surgery within two years: Abdominal surgery is the primary cause of small bowel obstruction. Based on medical literature, the expected rate of repeat surgery after SBO surgery is 30% without therapy; repeat surgeries generally start within the first two years.

Repeat Surgeries with CPA Therapy

Dataset #1 – Initial Data

Repeat surgeries up to five years after therapy: Initial clinical data examines our first 69 Clear Passage bowel obstruction patients for up to five years (mean 2.2 years) after therapy in two areas:

• Repeat surgeries with and without compliance with our home program

• Conditions where we observed negative outcomes

In this Dataset, 7% of patients we treated who followed our home program required additional surgery after therapy – much better than the 30% rate without Clear Passage therapy. In examining the unsuccessful cases, we were able to identify factors that pre-dispose a person to negative outcomes – to improve our results.

While our initial results with therapy were several times better than surgery, we continued to improve upon them over the years, as we modified our therapy, introduced a home maintenance program, and screened better for patients we felt would not benefit from our treatment.

Dataset #2 – Published Results

Repeat surgeries after therapy:

As our inquiries became more scientific, we created and published a validated test to get a broader view of our results. This test gave more definitive scientific results, which were published in the medical textbook "Intussusception and Bowel Obstruction" (Rice & King, 2015). This Dataset showed a 3% return for surgery in bowel obstruction patients up to 35 months (mean 19 months) after therapy. Based on medical literature, the expected rate for return surgery would have been 30% after 24 months – ten times our number.

Conclusion: A Chance to Avoid Surgery

Whether our "return to surgery" rate is 7% or 3% or between the two, it is clear that we greatly improved on the 30% "surgical return rate" for patients who do

not receive our therapy. As we near the end of our
first decade of treating patients with recurring bowel
obstructions, we assume our rates will remain stable —
or improve.

Pre-Disposing Factors for Poor Results

Over the years, we have learned to screen for conditions
that pre-dispose a person to negative results. Thus,
we now examine each patient's medical history for
present or past conditions that could lead to negative
outcomes, e.g. active infection, radiation enteritis (bowel
inflammation due to radiation therapy for cancer) and
uncontrolled inflammatory processes (e.g. Crohn's
disease uncontrolled by medication). To help our patients,
we now delay or decline applicants with conditions that
could lead to negative outcomes. Please consult us if you
have concerns about possible contraindications.

Life After Therapy

If you have undergone bowel obstruction surgery, your
intestines have been structurally compromised. It is
impossible to return the internal abdominal structure you
had before your first surgery. We cannot guarantee you
will be able to eat all of the foods you ate before your
began having obstructions. Some patients do; some do
not.

Nevertheless, it is clear from the numbers above, and
responses from the 400+ SBO patients we have treated

to date, that the benefits of therapy and our home maintenance program are significant for most Clear Passage patients. The success rates of our therapy in eliminating the need for surgery and restoring overall quality of life in our patients are very encouraging.

Future Studies

We continue to follow our patients over time and collect outcome data, both long term and immediately following treatment. It is worthy to note that the initial results from the many patients for whom we are presently gathering follow-up are equal or better than the numbers in the 69 patients we first treated.

Pelvic Pain and Sexual Dysfunction

Pelvic Pain and Sexual Dysfunction Improvements - General Population

Results:

Sexual Function and Pain Level Improvements – General (published in 2004)

96% reported reduced sexual intercourse pain (22/23)

56% reported improved or first-time orgasms (13/23)

78% reported greater or renewed desire (18/23)

65% reported increased satisfaction (15/23)

70% reported increased lubrication (16/23)

74% reported increased arousal (17/23)

91% reported overall increased sexual function (21/23 patients)

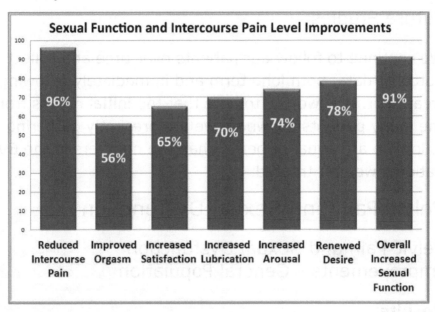

Medscape General Medicine – 2004

Increasing Orgasm and Decreasing Dyspareunia (Painful Intercourse) by a Manual Physical Therapy Technique

The first major study on our work treating pelvic pain and sexual dysfunction was published in 2004. We were honored that this study (data above) was published in *Medscape General Medicine*, owned by WebMD. At the time, it was the largest medical journal in the world, accessible to physicians in 237 countries. The editor was George Lundberg, MD, who had been editor of the *Journal of the American Medical Association* for the prior 17 years.

This study assessed the improvements of intercourse pain and overall sexual function in women with a history of chronic pelvic pain. In this population, 96% of patients reported a decrease in intercourse pain after CPA treatment and 91% reported an increase in overall sexual function.

Endometriosis Pain - Overview

Endometriosis is a complex condition that contains both mechanical and hormonal elements. In this condition, endometrial tissue that is normally found in the lining of the uterus, and that should be expelled with every menstrual period, is found in the interstitial spaces of the body – between organs, muscles, nerves and bones. When a woman has a period, these endometrial implants swell, pulling on the adhesions that frequently form between the implants and the structure on which they reside. Besides infertility, the main concerns for women with endometriosis are

• moderate to severe period pain

• moderate to severe pain with intercourse

• decreases sexual function (e.g., desire, lubrication, orgasm)

CPA therapy has been studied in all of these areas. In all cases, the therapy is designed to decrease the cross-linking, the tiny but powerful white attachments shown in the drawing in the chapter covering endometriosis. Below is data on reversing pain and sexual dysfunction for women we treated with endometriosis.

Pelvic Pain and Sexual Function Improvements - Endometriosis

Results:

50% reported reduced ovulation pain (9/18)

61% reported reduced menstrual pain (11/18)

80% reported reduced intercourse pain (24/30)

64% reported improved, or first-time orgasms (9/14)

71% reported increased desire (10/14)

86% reported increased arousal (12/14)

79% reported increased lubrication (11/14)

71% reported increased satisfaction (10/14)

93% reported improved overall sexual function

A 2011 study in the *Journal of Endometriosis and Pelvic Pain Disorders* reported on the effects of CPA on women who had endometriosis, menstrual and intercourse pain, and sexual problems. This two-part study was retrospective for women with sexual pain and dysfunction, and prospective for a different group of women, who had menstrual and intercourse pain. A follow-up study published in the same journal (2014) reported the effects of the therapy lasted over a year – which is the same time-frame used to test the effectiveness of endometriosis surgery.

While these studies were relatively small, the results were substantial enough to be considered valid (called statistically significant) by the biostatistician. In the retrospective analysis CPA therapy showed statistically significant improvements (P=.001) for every domain of sexual function listed above, including dyspareunia [intercourse pain] (P>.001), measured by the Female Sexual Function Index test. In the prospective analysis, CPA therapy showed statistically significant improvements in pain levels during the menstrual cycle (P>.014), with dysmenorrhea [menstrual pain] (P=.008) and with dyspareunia [intercourse pain] (P=.001), using the Mankoski Pain Scale.

Endometriosis: Menstrual pain, intercourse pain, sexual function

Results:

80% of women reported a reduction in intercourse pain

93% of women reported improvements in overall sexual

function.

61% of women reported a reduction in menstrual pain

50% of women reported a reduction in ovulation pain

Journal of Endometriosis – 2011

Decreasing Dyspareunia and Dysmenorrhea in Women with Endometriosis via a Manual Physical Therapy: Results from Two Independent Studies

This study assessed pain in women with endometriosis after treatment with the Wurn Technique. 61% of women in this study reported a reduction in menstrual pain and 80% reported a decrease in intercourse pain. Additionally, patients reported improvements in female sexual function, with 93% reporting improvements in overall sexual function.

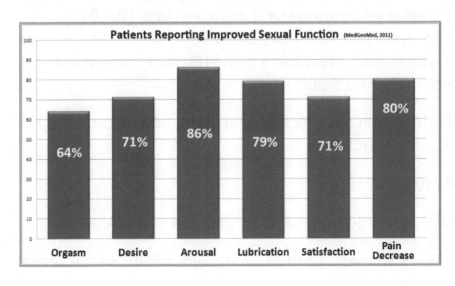

We tracked pain relief for one year, to compare with studies on surgical success rates. Results show success rates with this therapy are comparable to surgery (no better, and no worse), but without surgical risks, including of post-surgical adhesions.

Studies were published in the *Journal of Endometriosis*, 2011 (initial study) and 2014 (one year follow-up)

Statistical study data: Female Sexual Function Index (FSFI) Full Scale score showed overall statistically significant improvements (P=.001) for all domains of sexual function, including dyspareunia [intercourse pain] at (P>.001) in the retrospective analyses. Measured via the Mankoski Pain Scale, statistically significant improvements were noted in menstrual cycle (P>.014), dysmenorrhea (P=.008) and dyspareunia (P=.001) in the prospective analyses.

Made in United States
Troutdale, OR
04/26/2024

19467790R00090